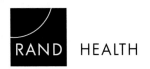

HEALTH

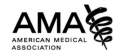

AMERICAN MEDICAL
ASSOCIATION

Effects of Health Care Payment Models on Physician Practice in the United States

The RAND Corporation

Mark W. Friedberg, Peggy G. Chen, Chapin White, Olivia Jung,

Laura Raaen, Samuel Hirshman, Emily Hoch, Clare Stevens

University of Southern California and The RAND Corporation

Paul B. Ginsburg

Weill Cornell Medical College

Lawrence P. Casalino

American Medical Association

Michael Tutty, Carol Vargo, Lisa Lipinski

Sponsored by the American Medical Association

For more information on this publication, visit www.rand.org/t/rr869

Library of Congress Control Number: 2015935308
ISBN: 978-0-8330-8894-9

Published by the RAND Corporation, Santa Monica, Calif.
© Copyright 2015 RAND Corporation
RAND® is a registered trademark.

www.rand.org

Preface

A variety of forces, including increasing health care costs and the passage of the Patient Protection and Affordable Care Act (Pub. L. 111-148, 2010), have led providers and payers to experiment increasingly with payment models other than fee for service. However, the ways in which practices respond and adapt to these payment models, creating their ultimate effects on individual physicians and allied health professionals, is unclear.

The project reported here, sponsored by the American Medical Association (AMA), aimed to describe the effects that alternative health care payment models (i.e., models other than fee-for-service payment) have on physicians and physician practices in the United States. These payment models included capitation, episode-based and bundled payment, shared savings, pay for performance, and retainer-based practice. Accountable care organizations and medical homes, which are two recently expanding practice and organization models that feature combinations of these alternative payment models, were also included. Project findings are intended to help guide efforts by the AMA and other stakeholders to make improvements to current and future alternative payment programs and help physician practices succeed in these new payment models.

The project began on February 4, 2014, and was completed on March 2, 2015. An advisory committee convened by the AMA provided input on key study activities, including project design, data collection methods, and interpretation of results. Committee membership is listed in Appendix A.

This work was sponsored by the AMA. The research was conducted in RAND Health, a division of the RAND Corporation. A profile of RAND Health, abstracts of publications, and ordering information can be found at www.rand.org/health.

Contents

Figure and Tables

Figure

Tables

Summary

Purpose

The project reported here, sponsored by the American Medical Association (AMA), aimed to describe the effects that alternative health care payment models (i.e., models other than fee-for-service payment) have on physicians and physician practices in the United States. These payment models included capitation, episode-based and bundled payment, shared savings, pay for performance (PFP), and retainer-based practice. Accountable care organizations and medical homes, which are two recently expanding practice and organizational models that are based on one or more of these alternative payment models, were also included. Project findings are intended to help guide efforts by the AMA and other stakeholders to make improvements to current and future alternative payment programs and help physician practices succeed in these new payment models—i.e., to help practices simultaneously improve patient care, preserve or enhance physician professional satisfaction, satisfy multiple external stakeholders, and maintain economic viability as businesses.

Methods

To describe the effects that payment programs have on physician practices, this project employed qualitative methods, incorporating multiple case studies, with each of 34 physician practices constituting a "case." Because the project sought to incorporate contextual information on market-level characteristics that might affect how practices respond to alternative payment models (e.g., the mix of competitors, health plans, and payment programs operating in the geographic area served by each practice), these 34 cases were nested within six geographically defined health care markets in the United States. Thus, within each market, we gathered data from physician practices and other market participants and observers: leaders of health plans and hospitals operating in the market, state or county medical societies, and state Medical Group Management Association (MGMA) chapters.

Main Findings

Effects of Payment Models at the Organizational Level
Changes in Organizational Structure
Multiple practice leaders and market interviewees reported that their own practices or others in their markets were changing their organizational models—predominantly by affiliating or

merging with other physician practices or aligning with or becoming owned by hospitals—in response to new payment models. From the practice leader perspective, the most prominent payment model–related reasons for these mergers were to enhance practices' ability to make the capital investments required to succeed in certain alternative payment models (especially investments in computers and data infrastructure), to negotiate contracts with health plans (including which performance measures and targets would be included), and to gain a sense of "safety in numbers." Leaders and physicians in multiple practices described uncertainty about how they would fare in alternative payment programs (and how such programs might evolve over time). For some of these practices, joining with a larger organization was seen as providing a general sense of security, no matter what payment programs might be introduced.

The reported effects of alternative payment models on practice stability, including overall financial impact, ranged from neutral to positive. No practice in our sample indicated experiencing major financial hardship as a result of new payment models. The retainer-based practices in our sample were small, and their physician-owners described their conversions to retainer-based payment as enabling an escape from market pressures that might otherwise have led to merger with other practices or early retirement.

Changes in Practice Operations

Respondents to our study perceived that alternative payment models have encouraged the development of team approaches to care management, featuring prominent roles for allied health professionals. In primary care practices in particular, physicians and practice leaders described appreciating how medical home programs and shared savings models (based on virtual global capitation) had allowed them to fund care manager positions. These dedicated care managers, who were allied health professionals in all cases in our sample, could concentrate on patient management between office visits, alleviating some of the pressure that physicians would feel if these activities were added to already-packed visits.

Alternative payment models that incentivize containment of total costs of care also increased the importance of offering expanded options for patients to access care from physician practices. Two examples of such expanded access were communication options for after-hours care (via web portal or telephone) and provision of in-person care in the community, outside the office.

Because global capitation and related shared savings models focus predominantly on primary care services for patient attribution and performance measurement, market observers and physician practices reported that these alternative payment models were changing relationships between primary care and subspecialist physicians. In some cases, these changes were collaborative, with multispecialty teams working to prevent progression of disease, without necessarily changing referral patterns. In other cases, changes in referral relationships were prominent, especially when alternative payment models led practices to reduce "leakage" to subspecialists in other organizations.

Increased Importance of Data and Data Analysis

In response to alternative payment models, physician practices reported making significant investments in their data management capabilities, ranging from adopting or upgrading electronic health records (EHRs) to committing physician and staff time and effort to data entry, management, and analysis. Several practices lacked in-house data management expertise and therefore invested in new types of staff dedicated to data management. Such investments were almost uniformly reported as being critical to practices' ability to succeed in these payment models.

In practices with more–highly developed data management capabilities, several leaders and physicians reported lacking the timely, accurate data they needed to respond to alternative payment models effectively. When present, these data deficiencies were a source of considerable frustration. The greatest concerns about data centered on the potential mismatch between data internal to a practice, from the EHR, reflecting "what actually happened" to the patient, and reports based on claims data, reflecting what was documented for billing purposes. Sometimes data in an EHR were not entered in a manner that facilitated capture during the coding and billing process (e.g., in free text rather than defined fields). Overall, practices seemed to trust their own internal EHR data more than they trusted external data, which they felt were at least one step removed from the "source of truth."

Finally, respondents noted that accurate price data for health care services and commodities (e.g., specialty drugs) could be difficult to obtain. When data on prices were unavailable, this limited practices' abilities to contain the costs of care—as encouraged in alternative payment models, such as capitation, shared savings, and episode-based and bundled payments.

Interactions Among Payment Programs and Between Payment Programs and Government Regulations

The multiplicity of PFP and other incentive programs has created a heavy administrative burden for some physician practices. Merely keeping track of payment program details, which vary from payer to payer, required management effort that might exceed the capacity of some practices. In response, larger physician practices and hospital systems have stepped into the role of boiling those incentives down into something that is more manageable, and palatable, for their physicians.

Performance incentives offered by multiple payers can reinforce each other, and incentives from one payer, in some cases, led to practice-wide changes affecting all of the practice's patients. But, a serious tension could also arise when practices participated in a mix of both fee-for-service (FFS) and risk-based contracts. In those situations, some practices reported facing fundamentally conflicting incentives—to increase volume under the FFS contract while reducing costs under the risk-based contract. This conflict was especially acute for hospital-owned physician practices, in which reductions in hospital utilization—which are strongly incentivized under risk-based contracts—could undermine the financial well-being of the parent organization.

In addition, multiple practices described spillover effects from the EHR installations and upgrades encouraged by meaningful-use incentives. In some cases, EHRs had positive effects, facilitating the achievement of performance targets in PFP and shared savings programs. In other cases, especially when customized EHR modifications tailored to an alternative payment model could not be transferred to a new EHR, some interviewees described significant setbacks in their ability to meet the goals of these alternative payment models.

Effects of Payment Models at the Individual Physician Level
Physician Incentives and Compensation

In general, we found that the financial incentives applied to physician practices via alternative payment models were not simply "passed through" to individual physicians. Even practices of relatively modest size reported shielding their physicians from direct exposure to the financial incentives created by payers—except in the case of traditional FFS payment. In fact, the greatest marginal financial incentive facing nearly all physicians in the study, even those in practices with substantial exposure to payment models intended to contain the costs of care (capitation, shared savings, and episode-based payment), was to increase "productivity" as measured by revenues or relative value units (RVUs), a unit of measurement for physician services originally created for Medicare FFS payment.

However, physician practices did not ignore the quality performance or cost-containment incentives they received from payers or seek to insulate individual physicians completely from making changes in response to practice-level financial incentives. Rather, practice leaders described transforming certain practice-level financial incentives (especially those concerning cost containment) into internal nonfinancial incentives for individual physicians, choosing instead to appeal to physicians' sense of professionalism, competitiveness, and desire to improve patient care. Common nonfinancial incentives included performance feedback and selectively retaining or terminating their physicians based on quality or efficiency performance.

In several practices, leaders acknowledged the presence of inconsistencies between financial and nonfinancial incentives (e.g., applying RVU-based financial incentives simultaneously with admonitions to contain costs). Reported barriers to achieving better alignment included a lack of alternatives to RVUs for measuring physician "productivity," a desire to avoid dramatic reallocation of income between physicians within the practice, and a need to balance the economic efficiency of physician compensation formulas with practical considerations (such as the operational costs of administering more-complex physician compensation formulas and the trade-off between the complexity and understandability of compensation incentives to physicians).

Generally speaking, alternative payment models had negligible effects on the aggregate income of individual physicians within our sample.

Some physicians reported wanting to have their incomes more closely linked to quality and efficiency of care. These physicians expressed an underlying desire to have better alignment between what they thought they should do for patients and what they were paid to do.

Physician Work and Professional Satisfaction

Within our sample, alternative payment models had not substantially changed how physicians delivered face-to-face patient care. However, the overall quantity and intensity of physician work had increased because of growing patient volume expectations and ongoing pressure for physicians to practice at the "top of license" (e.g., by delegating less intense patient encounters to allied health professionals), which was described as a potential contributor to burnout because lower-intensity patients could be an important source of respite for busy physicians.

Additional nonclinical work, particularly documentation requirements, created significant discontent. Physicians recognized the value of documentation tasks that were directly related to improvements in patient care, such as identifying patients with diabetes to facilitate better management of all patients with this condition, but they disliked the extra burden generated when documentation requirements were perceived as irrelevant to patient care.

Most physicians in practice leadership positions were optimistic and enthusiastic about alternative payment models, while most physicians not in leadership roles expressed at least some level of apprehension, particularly with regard to the documentation requirements of new payment models. Overall, even these physicians seemed to believe that major changes in payment methods would continue and acknowledged that some changes were useful. Nevertheless, their attitude was frequently one of resignation, rather than enthusiasm, because their day-to-day work life was more difficult and included burdens they did not believe would improve patient care.

Features of Payment Model Implementation
Factors Limiting the Effectiveness of New Payment Models as Implemented
Physicians and practice leaders described encountering three general types of operational problems in new payment programs that limited their effectiveness and sapped physicians' enthusiasm for them. By taking steps to avoid or prepare for these stumbling points, designers and implementers of future payment programs might be able to enhance their likelihood of achieving program goals.

First, physicians and practice leaders participating in a variety of alternative payment models described encountering errors in data integrity and timeliness, performance measure specification, and patient attribution (the process by which patients are assigned to a specific physician or practice). These payment models shared characteristics that might have made errors more likely: They were administratively more complex than FFS payment; some required payers to develop new measurement systems; and some were deployed for the first time quite quickly, without a "dress rehearsal" in which errors could be corrected before payments were on the line. Future participants in such models might consider such dress rehearsals or at least asking payers to design systems to quickly detect and correct implementation errors, which might be inevitable even in the best of cases.

Second, physicians had a variety of concerns about the implementation of performance and risk-adjustment measures underlying PFP, shared savings, and capitation programs. Broadly speaking, these concerns stemmed from a sense that the multiplicity of measures within and across programs could distract physician practices from making the changes to patient care that were actually the ultimate goal of many payment programs.

Third, the influence of uncontrollable, game-changing events in shared savings and capitation programs (e.g., the introduction of very high-cost specialty drugs) sapped physician practices' enthusiasm for these payment models. Finally, some physicians reported that they could not understand exactly what behaviors were being encouraged or discouraged by certain performance-based payment programs—even after seeking clarification from payers. Although these physicians reported that the performance bonuses they received were welcome, an incentive not understood by its target might not function as intended. Increasing the understandability of such incentive programs could enhance their effectiveness.

Conclusions

Nearly all physicians, physician practice leaders, and market observers who participated in this project described multiple simultaneous changes in payment models and regulations (such as meaningful use—a federal program to encourage physician practices to adopt and use EHRs). Most interviewees therefore described how interactions between these simultaneous changes, rather than the introduction of a given specific alternative payment model, affected physicians and physician practices. Prominent among these interactions were the tensions caused by lack of alignment among the plethora of performance measures and payment incentives deployed by different private and public payers.

Although our study did not seek explicitly to investigate the role of EHRs, the rapid uptake and upgrading of EHRs as a consequence of meaningful-use regulations was repeatedly described as the single greatest change in most practices, with both positive and negative spillover effects on nearly all practice efforts to respond to alternative payment models.

Physician practices played important roles as intermediaries and buffers between these changes in the health care marketplace and individual physicians within the practices. In some instances, practices magnified the impact that alternative payment models have on physicians' approaches to patient care—for example, by making substantial investments in new care pathways to enable successful performance in episode-based payment programs, even when such programs accounted for a negligible percentage of practice revenues. In other instances, practices shielded their physicians completely from specific aspects of alternative payment models—for example, when practice leaders made conscious decisions to ignore certain PFP measures to give their physicians a manageable array of targets for improvement. Physician practices also described translating external financial incentives from health plans into nonfinancial interventions (e.g., performance feedback and coaching) for individual physicians within the practice; this translation was nearly universal for financial incentives to contain the costs of care.

Practice leaders expressed considerable uncertainty about best strategies for responding to the combinations of alternative payment models that they faced, and doubts about the future compounded these uncertainties. Guided by practical limits on available capital and how much change their physicians could absorb quickly (especially when "change" amounted to "more work for each physician"), practice leaders tended to proceed cautiously, prioritizing areas in which multiple payment incentives overlapped with each other and with practices' internal priorities. For some smaller, independent practices, merging with larger practices or hospitals was an attractive option for accessing the capital necessary to succeed in alternative payment models (and for complying with new regulations, such as meaningful use) and enhancing their ability to control what alternative payment models they faced and how these would affect their physicians.

Implications

Informed by their experiences with alternative payment models, physicians, practice leaders, and other market observers described ways to enhance physician practices' abilities to respond successfully:

- **Physician practices need support and guidance to optimize the quantity and content of physician work under alternative payment models.** Alternative payment programs could create opportunities to reallocate physician work toward more satisfying content, which also could produce better, more efficient patient care. However, such payment programs also carry the risk of simply adding more work for already-overburdened physicians, risking burnout especially when such work is perceived as unrelated to good patient care. Developing physician leadership could help guide practices and health systems in their efforts to succeed in alternative payment models while preserving or enhancing physicians' professional satisfaction.
- **Addressing physicians' concerns about the operational details of alternative payment models could improve their effectiveness.** Although physician practices reported

these problems in a minority of cases, failure to execute payment programs as intended, use of clinical performance measures with unclear validity, and deployment of financial incentives that physicians do not understand can all undermine the effectiveness of alternative payment models. Health plans can anticipate and correct these problems by conducting dry runs of alternative payment programs before "going live" and clearly communicating their intent to physicians (i.e., communicating what, if anything, physicians should do differently in response to the program). If a program's specific intent cannot be communicated clearly, this could be a sign that the program should be redesigned.

- **To succeed in alternative payment models, physician practices need data and resources for data management and analysis.** Practices must make substantial data infrastructure investments to manage patient care effectively and monitor the performance measures that underlie many alternative payment programs. Although the financial resources necessary to make these investments can come from practices merging with each other and with hospitals, health plans also should consider investing in physician practices' data management capabilities. Such investments could enhance the effectiveness of alternative payment models. In addition, greater data sharing with physician practices (particularly sharing the prices of all health care services, including drugs) would help practices make the best possible use of their data management infrastructure.

- **Harmonizing key components of alternative payment models, especially performance measures, would help physician practices respond constructively.** Within the bounds of antitrust law, steps by health plans to align their payment models with each other will free up the substantial physician practice resources currently spent on wrangling hundreds of performance measures and trying to create a coherent response to the problem of "50 people shouting their priorities at you." If this cacophony can be ameliorated—and especially if government regulations can be harmonized with alternative payment models—practice leaders can better devote their attention to the difficult work of making meaningful and beneficial changes to their processes for patient care.

Acknowledgments

We gratefully acknowledge the invaluable time, expertise, and knowledge generously contributed by leaders and physicians in the physician practices, leaders of state and county medical societies, Medical Group Management Association chapters, health plans, and hospitals that participated in this study.

In addition, we gratefully acknowledge the following individuals who provided input into the contents of this report: Christine Sinsky, American Medical Association; Kenneth J. Sharigian, American Medical Association; J. James Rohack, Baylor Scott and White Health; John E. Billi, University of Michigan Medical School; Thomas J. Curry, Washington State Medical Association; Carolyn M. Clancy, U.S. Department of Veterans Affairs; Richard E. Wesslund, BDC Advisors; Nicholas Wolter, Billings Clinic; Susan L. Turney, Marshfield Clinic Health System; Gerald A. Maccioli, American Anesthesiology of North Carolina; Shawna Beck-Sullivan, RAND; Lori Uscher-Pines, RAND; and Robert A. Berenson, Urban Institute.

We also thank F. Jay Crosson, formerly of the American Medical Association, for his role in devising the project. We thank Kevin Spencer and David N. Gans of the Medical Group Management Association for advice on construction of the physician practice financial questionnaire.

Abbreviations

ACA	Patient Protection and Affordable Care Act
ACO	accountable care organization
AHRQ	Agency for Healthcare Research and Quality
AMA	American Medical Association
BPCI	Bundled Payments for Care Improvement
CEO	chief executive officer
CHF	congestive heart failure
CMS	Centers for Medicare and Medicaid Services
CPT	Current Procedural Terminology
CTS	Community Tracking Study
CTS-PS	Community Tracking Study Physician Survey
EHR	electronic health record
EMR	electronic medical record
FFS	fee for service
HEDIS	Healthcare Effectiveness Data and Information Set
HMO	health maintenance organization
HTPS	Health Tracking Physician Survey
IHA	Integrated Healthcare Association
IPA	independent practice association
IT	information technology
MA	medical assistant
MGMA	Medical Group Management Association
NCQA	National Committee for Quality Assurance

NSPO   National Study of Physician Organizations

PFP   pay for performance

PGP   Physician Group Practice

PHO   physician–hospital organization

PPO   preferred-provider organization

PQRS   Physician Quality Reporting System

PVBPM   Physician Value-Based Payment Modifier

QI   quality improvement

RVU   relative value unit

CHAPTER ONE

Introduction

The project reported here, sponsored by the American Medical Association (AMA), aimed to describe the effects of alternative health care payment models (i.e., models other than fee-for-service [FFS] payment) on physicians and physician practices in the United States. These payment models included capitation, episode-based and bundled payment, shared savings, pay for performance (PFP), and retainer-based practice. Accountable care organizations (ACOs) and medical homes, which are two recently expanding practice and organizational models that feature combinations of these alternative payment models, were also included. Project findings are intended to help guide efforts by the AMA and other stakeholders to make improvements to current and future alternative payment programs and help physician practices succeed in these new payment models.

The project began on February 4, 2014, and was completed on March 2, 2015. An advisory committee convened by the AMA provided input on key study activities, including project design, data collection methods, and interpretation of results. Committee membership is listed in Appendix A.

Organization of This Report

The report begins with the presentation and discussion of the conceptual model, which was used to organize the study.

Chapter Two on the conceptual model begins Part One and is followed by a background section in Chapter Three, which includes definitions of key alternative payment models and a review of the literature describing their effects. Chapter Four describes our methods, analysis, and limitations.

In Part Two, we describe our results:

- effects of payment models at the organizational level
  - changes in organizational structure (Chapter Five)
  - changes in practice operations (Chapter Six)
  - increased importance of data and data analysis (Chapter Seven)
  - interactions among payment programs and between payment programs and government regulations (Chapter Eight)
- effects of payment models at the individual physician level
  - physician incentives and compensation (Chapter Nine)
  - physician work and professional satisfaction (Chapter Ten)

- features of payment model implementation
  - factors limiting the effectiveness of new payment models as implemented (Chapter Eleven).

Each chapter gives an overview of findings, presents detailed qualitative results with illustrative participant quotes, and concludes with a brief review of relationships between study findings and previously published research. The chapters are written so that they can be read independently and in any order. Because of the overlapping nature of the topics in this report, some findings appear in more than one chapter.

Finally, in the conclusion in Chapter Twelve, we present recommendations for the future, characterized as challenges and opportunities. We also provide two appendixes. Appendix A, provided here, lists the committee members. Appendix B, available online, reproduces the interview guides.

PART ONE

Model, Background, and Methods

The following chapters present the purpose, conceptual model, definitions, and methods underlying our study, as well as a review of previously published literature relevant to the study.

Conceptual Model

Our conceptual model, which was informed by our review of the literature (in Chapter Three) and the data analyses described in Chapter Four, seeks to describe and categorize potential relationships between the design of a given payment model, how this payment model could interact with physician practice characteristics and other payment models applied to the practice, and outcomes of these interactions—which include effects on practices, physicians, and patients. This conceptual model was meant to both guide data collection and be informed and improved by study findings.

As displayed in the conceptual model (Figure 2.1), a payment model is defined by its characteristics in four categories: the basis of payment, the rate of payment, other design details, and the role of chance. It is possible for a single payment model to have multiple characteristics in each of these categories. Elements in the first three of these categories typically are spelled out in a contract (or, for government payers, regulation) between a payer and a physician practice.

The role of chance, which is the degree to which payment amounts are determined by luck (i.e., because of random variation in measures of the costs or quality of care), is rarely spelled out explicitly in payment contracts. However, the role of chance is still determined in part by contract provisions and therefore is considered a characteristic of the payment model. For example, performance measures based on small numbers of patients might have low reliability, thereby increasing the degree to which payments based on these measures occur at random.

These design elements of each payment model then interact with physician practice characteristics and other payment models to which a given physician practice is exposed to produce the following categories of outcomes, each of which constitutes an area of interest for the current study:

- incentives and interventions to affect individual physician decisionmaking: financial and nonfinancial incentives, other types of interventions, and organizational units to which incentives are applied
- changes in practice goals, including changes intended and not intended to affect patient care (i.e., the mix of services the practice intends to produce)
- changes in the production model for patient care: changes in the mix and composition of labor and capital
- organizational changes: sustainment or changes of practice model (e.g., ownership), whether the practice continues or ends as a business
- physician outcomes: work quantity and content, professional satisfaction, and compensation in aggregate and per unit of work.

**Figure 2.1
Conceptual Model**

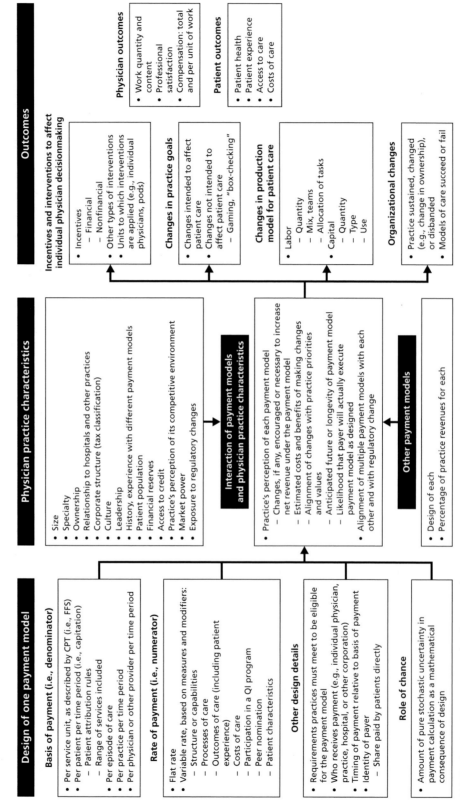

NOTE: CPT® = Current Procedural Terminology. CPT® is a registered trademark of the AMA. QI = quality improvement.

RAND *RR869-2.1*

Patient outcomes, although constituting a critically important set of outcomes of payment models, are outside the scope of the current study, except insofar as patient outcomes could affect physicians and physician practices (e.g., by triggering PFP payments).

CHAPTER THREE

Background: Scan of the Literature on Effects of Payment Models on Physician Practice

Overview

A variety of forces, including increasing health care costs and the passage of the Patient Protection and Affordable Care Act (ACA), have led providers and payers (both private and public sector) to experiment increasingly with payment models other than simple FFS. These expanding models include global payments, shared savings (e.g., ACOs), physician–hospital gainsharing, episode-based payments, PFP, and subscription or retainer arrangements and are frequently coupled with new practice organizational forms, such as medical homes and ACOs (Schneider, Hussey, and Schnyer, 2011). However, the ways in which practices respond and adapt to these payment models, creating their ultimate effects on individual physicians and allied health professionals, is unclear. Similarly, the extent to which these currently expanding payment models motivate physician practices to change their business strategies (e.g., by merging with each other or affiliating with hospitals) is unknown.

Two prior, long-running studies have been particularly notable for their focus on payment models and organizational characteristics of physician practices. The first is the National Study of Physician Organizations (NSPO), a series of three surveys of physician practice administrative leaders conducted in 2000–2001, 2006–2007, and 2011–2012. In the past decade, the NSPO has contributed valuable insights on the prevalence and relationships between payment models, structural capabilities, and other practice characteristics in the United States (Robinson, Shortell, Li, et al., 2004). However, the NSPO has not collected data from individual physicians working within the surveyed practices that would allow description of relationships between payment models, physician work content, and other aspects of the patient care experience.

The second major study was the Community Tracking Study (CTS) Physician Survey (CTS-PS) and Health Tracking Physician Survey (HTPS), conducted by the Center for Studying Health System Change. The CTS and HTPS surveyed physicians in five waves (with some design modifications over time) between 1997 and 2008. The community-level component of the CTS collected qualitative data from a diverse set of 12 health care markets in the United States between 1997 and 2010, establishing a valuable baseline for understanding the evolution of these markets (and, by extrapolation, the U.S. health care system more broadly) leading up to the expansion of newer payment and organizational models, such as ACOs and medical homes. However, the CTS and HTPS have not surveyed physicians since 2008, and the study will not be repeated by the Center for Studying Health System Change, which merged with Mathematica Policy Research at the end of 2013.

In addition to these two major studies, recent evaluations of novel commercial payment models, such as the Alternative Quality Contract of Blue Cross Blue Shield of Massachusetts, have focused on effects on patient care (finding, for example, that, under shared savings, practices have redirected referrals to lower-cost settings) but have not assessed physician work experience or practice financial sustainability (Mechanic, Santos, et al., 2011).

Although evaluations of new Medicare payment pilots are under way, to our knowledge, there are no current efforts to describe the scope of new payment models promulgated by private payers or to investigate how physician practices are responding to simultaneous, potentially conflicting payment models from private and public payers. Therefore, there is an unmet need to describe the effects that current combinations of rapidly changing private and public payment models are having on physicians' practices, professional lives, and delivery of patient care—and to explore how these effects are modified by market context.

Payment Models Included in the Scan

In this section, we define the key types of payment models covered in this literature scan, using the project's conceptual model as a framework. We include the following categories of payment models. First, three "underlying" payment models can exist alone, without other types of payment: FFS, capitation, and episode-based payment. Second, we include PFP and shared savings as "supplementary" payment models that can coexist with one or more underlying payment models (but cannot exist on their own without underlying payment models). Third, we include retainer-based payment models as variations of capitation in which the patient typically pays a fee in exchange for access to a physician practice.

With the exception of retainer-based practices, we do not investigate the role of copayments, deductibles, or other payments that patients could be required to make to physician practices. Though patients' direct payment responsibilities could affect physician practices in many ways, this aspect of benefit design (which can coexist with any underlying payment model) is outside the scope of this report.

Fee for Service

In simple FFS payment models, the basis of payment is per service unit, usually following service unit descriptions in the CPT codes. For a given provider, the rate of payment is a flat rate per service unit; i.e., all services of a given type are paid the same piece rate. Other design details could vary considerably, with different entry requirements and shares of payment for which patients are responsible (e.g., deductibles and copayment amounts). Typically, practices are paid on a rolling basis, after billing for each service unit they provide to patients. In theory, there is no role of chance in calculating FFS payment amounts: As soon as an FFS contract is signed, the amount of payment for a given service unit can be known with certainty (although practices can still be uncertain about payment amounts when FFS contracts lack clear and complete payment information).

Capitation

In capitation models, the basis of payment is per patient per time period, with the time period typically being one month. To decide which patients are included for a given physician practice, attribution rules must be applied. In managed care plans, a common attribution rule would be to attribute a patient to a primary care physician when the patient explicitly identifies to the payer his or her choice of primary care physician. When patients do not identify their physicians, other attribution rules can be applied, ranging from "contact capitation" for subspecialists (in which seeing a patient once results in a capitation payment for services in that subspecialty) to more-complex attribution rules, such as those based on providing the plurality or majority of qualifying services. For a given attributed patient, capitation models can include all services the patient receives during the contracted time period or only a subset of these services (e.g., a primary care practice could have a capitation contract that covers only the professional fees for primary care services). The rate of payment could vary based on patient characteristics, such as age, sex, and health status, typically with higher rates for patients whose care is expected to be more expensive during the time period of the contract. The rate of payment might or might not be intended to fully cover patients' expected costs of care.

Other design details can vary. Notably, in concept, payment can occur at any time following patient attribution; it is not necessary to wait until the end of the time period of the contract. For example, practices in a yearlong capitation contract might be paid for each patient on a monthly basis.

In pure capitation, there is no role of chance in the amount of payment per patient per time period: As soon as a capitation contract is signed, the amount of payment for a given patient per time period is known with certainty. Of course, physician practices receiving capitation payments could be taking considerable financial risks—but the random component is confined to the costs of delivering care (which is distinct from the amount of payment received). On the other hand, if capitation contracts include risk-sharing, in which the physician practice is partially insured by the health plan against unexpectedly high costs of care, the amount of payment could be partially determined by random variation but in a way that reduces a practice's financial risk.

Episode-Based and Bundled Payments

As their name implies, episode-based payment models use episodes of care as the bases of payment. Episodes can be defined in multiple ways, typically according to a set of diagnoses and services provided over a specified time frame. For example, an episode of care could include an inpatient hospital stay plus all services provided during a window surrounding the inpatient stay.

When episode-based payments cover the services of multiple providers involved in the episode, such as different physician specialties, hospital care, and post–acute care, these payment models are called *bundled* payments. For a given episode type, the rate of payment can be flat or variable—but because the intent of such models is to give physician practices an incentive to contain the costs of care, the rate of payment typically does not increase if costs of care are higher. Payment can occur before, during, or after an episode of care.

As with capitation, the role of chance in episode-based payment models can vary. The amount of payment per episode can be prespecified in a contract (leaving no random component) or include risk-sharing to insure the practice against very high episode costs (resulting in random variation in the payment amount). Also as with capitation, episode-based payments expose physician practices to random variation in the costs of delivering care within an episode.

Supplementary Payment Models

As explained above, the payment models detailed in this section (PFP and shared savings) cannot exist on their own and must be coupled with one of the three underlying payment models (FFS, capitation, or episode-based payment). In this section, we also discuss retainer-based payment models, a variant of capitation that frequently coexists with FFS.

Pay for Performance

In PFP models, the basis of payment can vary widely, including all options listed in the conceptual model. The rate of payment is variable, with amounts determined by the measures and modifiers listed in the conceptual model. For example, a per-patient bonus could be paid at the end of a year if and only if the practice exceeds certain performance thresholds on measures of quality, with higher bonuses for medically complex patients. PFP payments also can be based on measures of costs or utilization of care, blurring the distinction between PFP and shared savings. The timing of payment must follow the measurement on which the payment rate is based, but other design details could also vary. For example, PFP bonuses or penalties can be paid via changes in underlying FFS payment rates in subsequent contract years, rather than lump-sum payments. The role of chance in determining PFP payments could be significant, especially when there is large random variation in the measurement underlying the calculation of the payment rate (e.g., when sample sizes are small). PFP payments could be calculated for and paid to individual clinicians, practices, or organizations that include multiple practices (e.g., independent practice associations [IPAs]).

Shared Savings

In shared savings models, which are added to an underlying chassis of FFS payment (i.e., FFS persists as the main day-to-day payment method), the basis of payment is per patient per time period, as in capitation models, or per episode of care, as in episode-based payment models.

Variants of capitation can be operationalized through shared savings contracts. In such virtual-capitation models, practices are paid FFS throughout the contract year, rather than receiving capitation payments before or during the year. At the end of the year, total costs of care for the attributed patient population are compared to a cost target (the virtual-capitation amount for the population), triggering a lump-sum bonus or penalty. This cost target can be calculated many ways; two common variants are (1) historical costs of care for the physician practice and (2) expected costs for patients in the community served by the physician practice (i.e., taking an average that includes other providers also serving the community).

Unlike pure capitation, the virtual-capitation rate of payment is variable: a share of the observed savings relative to the cost target. The percentage of observed savings that is shared can be determined by performance on various measures in addition to costs of care, incorporating an element of PFP. Some, but not all, shared savings contracts feature downside risk for physician practices, in which the practice pays a financial penalty if actual costs exceed expected costs (i.e., the rate of payment to practices can take on negative values).

As in virtual capitation, shared savings can be used to operationalize virtual-episode models. In such models, practices are paid FFS during the time period of the contract (typically a year). Episodes are retroactively identified at the end of the year, and the average cost per episode among episodes attributed to a given provider is compared to a cost target (the virtual-episode payment amount), triggering a lump-sum bonus or penalty. Bonus amounts can also be based on factors beyond costs, such as measured quality.

Because actual costs must be calculated, the shared savings can be paid only after the time period of the contract has concluded. The role of chance in shared savings models can be significant, especially for smaller numbers of attributed patients.

Retainer-Based Payment

The defining feature of retainer payment models, also known as subscription or concierge models, is a capitation payment (typically per patient per year or per month; also known as a membership fee) that is typically paid from the patient to the physician practice directly. This capitation payment covers a defined range of services and can be supplemented by other payment arrangements, such as FFS, typically billed to the patient's insurance (separate from the capitation payment), for services not within the range covered by the capitation payment. For example, the capitation payment might cover services that are not included in typical FFS contracts (e.g., after-hours access to physicians via phone), with office visits paid via FFS. Or, a more inclusive capitation payment might cover all primary care services for a year (including but not limited to those defined by CPT codes), with no FFS component. In this inclusive case, when the capitation payment includes primary care services that a health plan typically would cover, the fee might be paid, in part or in full, by a third-party payer.

Importantly, the capitation fee in retainer payment models commonly also serves as an entry fee that allows access to further services, either free or paid à la carte, from the provider. Typically, there is no role of chance in determining the amount of the retainer fee for a given patient.

Organizational Models That Combine Payment Models

Using two new organizational models for physician practices—medical homes and ACOs—we illustrate how payment models can be combined in various ways. In this report, we conceptualize medical homes and ACOs as necessitating some kind of alternative payment model (i.e., we do not consider the case of a medical home or ACO that is paid under FFS exclusively).

Medical Homes

There are many definitions of medical homes and, correspondingly, many different models for paying medical homes (Edwards, Abrams, et al., 2014). In nearly all medical homes that are not part of larger organizations taking global capitation, the underlying chassis of FFS payment persists as the practice's main revenue source. However, medical home practices often receive additional payments in the form of higher FFS payment rates (enhanced FFS) or per-patient per-month fees, sometimes called care management or medical home payments, that are paid in addition to traditional FFS payments. Also, medical homes could receive PFP payments for performing well on measures of quality, patient experience, or costs and could be eligible to receive shared savings payments based on annual total costs of care for their patients (a form of virtual capitation, as discussed above).

In general, medical home pilots share the requirement that medical homes provide primary care services to their patients and feature a variable rate of payment that is based on practice structural capabilities. For example, this variable rate can be linked to National Committee for Quality Assurance (NCQA) recognition as a medical home and be paid as a monthly or yearly amount per patient (often called a care management fee) or per practice or physician (e.g., to offset costs of investing in medical home capabilities). But this variable rate also can be linked to other structural criteria (e.g., attainment of payer-specific medical home recognition) and be paid on other bases, such as enhanced FFS rates. In addition, other payment models not related to practice structure could also be present, including PFP (e.g., based on processes of care) and virtual-capitation models operationalized via shared savings. Finally, in nearly all medical homes that are not part of larger organizations taking global capitation, an underlying chassis of FFS payment persists as the practice's main revenue source.

The role of chance in determining payments to medical homes depends on the payment models included in a given medical home program. For example, payments to small practices (each with few patients) in a medical home program that includes PFP and shared savings could have large random components because of small sample sizes for measuring performance and costs of care.

Accountable Care Organizations

As with medical homes, there are many definitions of ACOs and multiple ways to pay an ACO. Broadly, ACOs are large health systems (that might or might not include a hospital) or collections of physician practices that jointly enter an ACO contract with a payer. In a Medicare ACO contract, an ACO is paid via FFS but can receive shared savings at the end of the year if it performs well on measures of quality and patient experience and holds the total costs for its population of attributed patients below a defined target (i.e., a form of virtual capitation). In private health plan ACO contracts, ACOs are often paid in this way as well, but, in some cases, the ACO is paid via capitation for professional services and is eligible for additional payments if it performs well on PFP measures or for shared savings. In these ACO payment models, the amount of shared savings bonus (i.e., percentage of savings paid to the ACO) also can vary based on the number of patients in the denominator. The bonus is typically paid as a lump sum for the previous year, but other bases of payment are possible (e.g., an "uplift" modification to the practice's FFS rates in the next contract year).

Alternative Payment Models: Existing Evidence on Prevalence and Effects on Physician Practice Outcomes

In this section, we present an overview of the published literature on each payment model in these categories:

- *prevalence:* We include historical and current estimates of the prevalence of the payment model.
- *incentives and interventions to affect individual physician decisionmaking:* We summarize relationships between how practices are paid (payment models) and how practices incentivize and influence their physicians.
- *organizational changes:* We present relationships between practice participation in payment models and changes to practice size, ownership, and affiliation with other organizations.

- *physician outcomes:* We review relationships between payment models and physician professional satisfaction, work quantity and content, and overall compensation.

Capitation
Prevalence

Despite being hailed as the "payment model of the future" (Gesensway, 1996), capitation has always been the exception rather than the norm. The spread of capitation use hit its peak around 1996–1997 when, according to the CTS-PS, more than half of physicians reported that their practices received at least some of their revenues in the form of capitation (Lake and St. Peter, 1997). At that time, some believed that capitation was widespread and on the verge of becoming the norm (Havighurst, 1999), while others thought that capitation was never that pervasive and "still an illusion for many" (Gesensway, 1996). Even during the height of its popularity in the mid-1990s, capitation was reported as a source of revenue for only about one-third of the multispecialty groups in the United States (Gesensway, 1996).

For office-based physician visits, the rate of capitation use peaked at around 16 percent in 1996–1998 and fell to around 7 percent in 2007 (Zuvekas and Cohen, 2010). The switch in focus from avoiding overutilization to ensuring that appropriate and needed services are provided also reinforced this downward trend (Robinson, 2001b).

The use of capitation varies geographically and by type of service. For example, capitation of primary care has historically been more common than for specialized care (Lake and St. Peter, 1997). A survey of medical groups and IPAs in California that used capitation to pay primary care physicians showed that payments were typically restricted to cover only primary care services (Rosenthal, Frank, et al., 2002).

Capitation has been, and continues to be, more prevalent on the West Coast (Lake and St. Peter, 1997; Zuvekas and Cohen, 2010). Other factors associated with participation in capitation contracts include whether physicians are salaried employees of a hospital (Ubokudom, 1998) and whether medical groups and IPAs are located in markets heavily penetrated by managed care (Robinson, Shortell, Li, et al., 2004).

In California in the late 1990s, many different forms of capitation were in use, ranging from capitation just for professional services to global capitation arrangements that included full risk for hospital services (Rosenthal, Frank, et al., 2002). Various forms of capitation have survived and are used today. A survey of large multispecialty medical groups participating in risk contracts, such as capitation, showed that, on average, around 25 percent of the respondents' patient care revenue came from global capitation contracts and 9 percent from partial capitation or shared-risk contracts (Mechanic and Zinner, 2012). In 2012, 35 percent of the commercially insured in Massachusetts were enrolled in plans that use either global payment or limited budget, which are two variants of capitation akin to global capitation and partial capitation described above (Center for Health Information and Analysis, 2013).

Effects of Capitation: Incentives and Interventions to Affect Individual Physician Decisionmaking

The key rationale for capitating physician payments is to create a financial incentive for physicians to provide lower-cost care. Global capitation—in which an integrated delivery system is responsible for all services or primary care physicians are held financially responsible for services provided by others—creates a further incentive for physicians to reduce unnecessary referrals, hospital admissions, and the ordering of prescriptions, tests, and so on.

Capitation payments to physician practices have some influence over compensation arrangements for individual physicians, but physician organizations heavily insulate individual physicians from the financial incentives to reduce services inherent in capitation (Rosenthal, Frank, et al., 2002).

One way capitation payment to practices affects individual physicians is by spurring a shift in compensation to salary plus bonus,[1] with bonus payments tied to performance goals for efficiency, patient satisfaction, committee service, and other productivity incentives (Glass, Pieper, and Berlin, 1999). Medical groups receiving capitation payments are more likely to use salary-based compensation arrangements with their physicians than they are to use productivity-based arrangements (Robinson, Casalino, et al., 2009). And, at the market level, medical groups and IPAs in markets with high levels of health maintenance organization (HMO) penetration have a higher likelihood of applying fixed compensation to their individual physicians—either salary or capitation payments—than of applying productivity-based compensation (Robinson, Shortell, Li, et al., 2004). However, many practices still use productivity, as measured by relative value units (RVUs), as the foundation for compensation.

Capitation can affect the pressures on physician behavior in two ways: In some cases, it creates pressure to reduce the number of services provided; in other cases, it alleviates the pressure to increase the number of services provided. According to the 2000–2001 CTS-PS, overall, only 7 percent of physicians reported a perceived incentive to reduce services provided to patients, but that share was higher among physicians in groups with larger shares of revenue from capitation (Reschovsky, Hadley, and Landon, 2006). Conversely, practice ownership, flexible compensation, and bonuses to employed physicians were associated in the 2004–2005 CTS-PS with perceived incentives to increase services (Landon, Reschovsky, Pham, et al., 2009). Similarly, among generalist physicians seeing managed care patients in three Minnesota health plans, those in more capitation-heavy practices were more likely to perceive pressure to limit referrals (Keating, Landon, et al., 2004).

Effects of Capitation: Organizational Changes

Physician practices that accept global capitation payments take on the role of managing insurance risk—the risk of an adverse event happening to a patient because of the patient's predisposition or random event (e.g., breaking a bone, getting in a car accident, or getting the flu)—in addition to providing clinical services (Hussey, Ridgely, and Rosenthal, 2011). The wave of bankruptcies of physician organizations and physician practice management companies in California in the late 1990s illustrates the risks in taking on that role—many practices were ill-prepared for the delegation of risk and medical management from health plans to physicians, coupled with cost increases due to policy changes mandating benefits and generous changes in health plan offerings (Fountain et al., 1999).

Historically, larger physician practices were more likely to participate in capitated contracts (American Medical Association Center for Health Policy Research, 1997). In a capitated environment, "information systems—and data analysis—are essential to long-term success," and practices that are paid through capitation report greater delegation to and reliance on support staff and information technology (IT) staff (Gans, 2013). These findings suggest that

---

[1]   Salary is not included as a payment model in this report because it is not available to the third-party payer; rather, salary can be instituted only by physician practices or other provider organizations that receive third-party payment and that then develop their own compensation approaches to their constituent physicians.

capitated payments could promote physicians joining into larger practices, but we did not identify any evidence in the literature to indicate whether capitation has actually spurred physician practices toward one particular model of organization over others. Discerning the direction of causation in this research area is challenging, especially in cross-sectional analyses, because both directions are plausible: Larger practices might be more likely to participate in capitation, or capitation could cause practices to grow in size.

Effects of Capitation: Physician Outcomes

The evidence on capitation's effect on physician professional satisfaction is mixed. In aggregate measures overall, physicians tended to express dissatisfaction with capitation: Studies found that physicians in states with high levels of penetration by HMOs were more likely to report dissatisfaction than in low-HMO-penetration states in 1995 (Donelan, 1997), staff- and group-model HMO physicians were less satisfied with their careers in medicine and articulated a greater likelihood of intending to leave their practices than physicians practicing in other settings were (Linzer, Konrad, et al., 2000), and almost 15 percent of generalist physicians seeing managed care patients in three Minnesota health plans also expressed dissatisfaction with their jobs (Keating, Landon, et al., 2004). Physicians' dissatisfaction with capitation was more pronounced than their dissatisfaction with FFS (Nadler et al., 1999). In a survey of almost 800 physicians with capitated contracts in California, physicians expressed lower satisfaction with their relationships with capitated patients, the quality of care they provided to capitated patients, the ability to treat capitated patients according to their own best judgment, and the ability to obtain specialty referrals in juxtaposition to patients under other coverage arrangements (Kerr et al., 1997).

Capitation in the 1990s has been characterized as "an economic success but a political failure" (Robinson, 2001a, p. 6). The concerns with capitation lie both in the ethical considerations and on the practical side. On the ethical side, "[c]apitation is an incentive to do less, an idea that troubles physicians and patients alike" (Morrison, 2000, p. 81). A systematic review identified possible risks from capitation and similar arrangements, including "limited continuity of care, . . . reduced range of services, . . . delayed treatment, [and] conflict of interests between the physician and the patient" (Chaix-Couturier et al., 2000, p. 135).

However, with particular features of capitation, especially those concerning administrative support, physicians expressed satisfaction. One survey of physicians practicing in HMOs in Massachusetts in 1997 demonstrated that physicians were satisfied with administrative processes (Linzer, Konrad, et al., 2000), and another survey of physicians practicing under a similar setting noted that physicians were satisfied with high quality, autonomy, leisure time, and experiencing fewer administrative hassles (Murray et al., 2001). Physicians belonging to a hospital organization at an urban teaching hospital expressed increased satisfaction with fully capitated contracts over time from 1996 to 1997—specifically, with patient load, time to discuss patient needs, and benefits of care coordination (Nadler et al., 1999).

Episode-Based and Bundled Payments
Prevalence

In the past three decades, the Medicare program has led the way in applying episode-based and bundled payments. Beginning in the 1980s, Medicare switched from reimbursing hospitals for their reasonable costs to paying a prospectively determined amount per inpatient stay, which treats the inpatient stay as an episode of care (Mayes and Berenson, 2006). Medicare has expanded episode-based payments to apply to a broader and broader range of services, including surgical care, hospital outpatient services (Wynn, 2005), and home health services (McCall et al., 2001). The last major holdouts in the Medicare program are within the physician fee schedule, in which, for services not included in an episode (i.e., most nonsurgical services), physicians continue to be paid separately for each patient encounter.

Centers for Medicare and Medicaid Services (CMS) has also conducted a series of large demonstration projects to test the bundling of payments for services provided by multiple types of providers, such as hospitals and physicians, who have historically been paid under separate systems. The pilots have been applied to several types of episodes, including cardiac bypass, cataract surgery, and joint-replacement surgeries (American Hospital Association, 2010; Cromwell et al., 2011; Nelson, 2012; CMS, 2013). Building on lessons learned from these demonstrations, CMS initiated the three-year Medicare Acute Care Episode demonstration in 2009, in which five participating organizations negotiated a global payment that was discounted from the standard payment for several cardiac and joint-replacement procedures (Calsyn and Emanuel, 2014). Most recently, in 2011, CMS began implementing the Bundled Payments for Care Improvement (BPCI) demonstrations as authorized under Section 3023 of the ACA. In January 2013, CMS selected health care organizations to participate in the demonstration that bundles payment for 48 episodes. Four different models are being tested over three years, including three types of retrospective episode models (acute-care hospital stay only, acute-care hospital stay plus post–acute care, and post–acute care only) and one prospective episode model for acute-care hospital stays only (CMS, 2014b). All of the BPCI bundles are centered on an inpatient hospital stay.

CMS's expansion of bundled payments has occurred alongside private-sector initiatives (Kary, 2013). In 2006, the first major private-sector bundled payment program was launched. The PROMETHEUS Payment model received funding from the Commonwealth Fund and Robert Wood Johnson Foundation to develop bundled payment systems at four initial pilot sites (Painter, 2012). Another key private-sector initiative is the Geisinger Health System ProvenCare bundled payment system for nonemergency coronary artery bypass graft procedures, which includes all preoperative care, hospital and professional fees, postdischarge care, and treatment for any complications that arise within 90 days of the surgery (Casale et al., 2007; Fangmeier, 2013).

A 2012 survey by Bailit Health Purchasing identified 19 nonfederal bundled payment programs, of which nine have fully operationalized at least one bundled payment, two are conducting observational studies with no payment involved, and eight are in the process of developing a bundled payment (Painter, 2012). Additionally, some large employers have formed bundled payment arrangements with medical providers for certain surgical procedures. For example, Lowe's has had a bundled payment program with the Cleveland Clinic for coronary artery bypass graft surgeries since 2010. Lowe's waives the $500 deductible for its employees and covers travel expenses to the Cleveland Clinic, which accepts a flat payment for the procedure and related services. Beginning in 2014, Lowe's and Walmart will use bundled payments for knee and hip replacements at four health systems (Fangmeier, 2013).

Although interest in bundled payment programs is high among private-sector payers, early adopters have faced significant, and sometimes insurmountable, hurdles. For example, three years after initiating a multisite pilot of the PROMETHEUS Payment model, none of the sites had executed a contract incorporating the new payment program (Hussey, Ridgely, and Rosenthal, 2011). Although leaders at the pilot sites believed in and were motivated to implement the payment model, they reported significant challenges, including defining the bundles in terms of which services are included or excluded, defining and agreeing on the payment method and amount of financial risk for providers and payers, implementing quality measurements to protect against unintended consequences, determining accountability for each episode of care because many providers might care for a patient, engaging providers to change care delivery, and redesigning care delivery to reduce costs and improve quality (Hussey, Ridgely, and Rosenthal, 2011). Similar organizational challenges appeared more recently in California in the Integrated Healthcare Association (IHA) bundled payment demonstration (Ridgely et al., 2014).

Effects of Episode-Based and Bundled Payments: Incentives and Interventions to Affect Individual Physician Decisionmaking

The rationale for episode-based payment is to give providers an incentive to reduce the intensity of services and the costs of treatment within each episode, and the evidence from the literature generally indicates that episode-based payments have been successful in reducing utilization (Hussey, Mulcahy, et al., 2012). It is not clear, however, what interventions have prompted physicians to shift to less-intensive treatment patterns. Geisinger's ProvenCare bundled payment initiative placed a heavy emphasis on building new workflows into electronic health records (EHRs) and providing real-time feedback to providers (Berry et al., 2009), but that system's approach and experience might not be typical.

However, there might be other changes in behavior in response to episode-based and bundled payments. The Acute Care Episode demonstration, which saved Medicare an average of $585 per episode (which fell to $319 saved per episode after administrative costs), observed that the greatest cost savings were earned from increased negotiations with suppliers to reduce the cost of materials and equipment (Urdapilleta et al., 2013)—suggesting that, within their practices, physicians were incentivized to use the same equipment (e.g., all using joint prostheses from the same vendor), increasing their bargaining leverage.

Effects of Episode-Based and Bundled Payments: Organizational Changes

Episode-based payments can significantly alter the relationships and balance of power among providers and between provider and payers. Concerns about these changes emerged 30 years ago in the context of episode-based payments for hospitals, which did not bundle together hospital and physician payments. For example, the introduction in 1983 of Medicare's bundled payments to hospitals created intense pressure on hospitals to reduce lengths of stay and treatment costs (Feder, Hadley, and Zuckerman, 1987). In 1985, Arnold Relman observed that

> the economic interests of the hospital and the doctor are now in opposition rather than in concert, at least with respect to Medicare patients. Physicians have always tended to be a little suspicious of hospital administrators, often regarding them as bureaucratic impediments to the achievement of optimal care. Such suspicions can only be exacerbated under the new payment system, which requires hospital management to press the medical staff for restraint in ordering elective and services and for earlier discharge of patients. (Relman, 1985, p. 108)

The pressure on hospitals to reduce lengths of stay has contributed to the proliferation of hospitalists (FOJP Service Corporation, 2013); hospitalists' role, in part, is to reduce inpatient lengths of stay, and there is evidence that they are somewhat effective in that role (Coffman and Rundall, 2005). Medicare's BPCI might further shift power and control toward hospitals because hospitals are the entities that will bear the financial risk for professional services and post–acute care services provided during episodes of care.

Pay for Performance

Prevalence

A decade ago, PFP was more of a buzzword than a reality. Since then, PFP has moved off the drawing board and into widespread practice (Bodenheimer et al., 2005). PFP is commonly applied in physician payment models, including among commercial health plans, Medicare, and state Medicaid plans. One key support for the spread of PFP models is the development of validated "off-the-shelf" quality measures, including Healthcare Effectiveness Data and Information Set (HEDIS) measures produced by NCQA, and other measures produced by the National Quality Forum and the Agency for Healthcare Research and Quality (AHRQ). PFP incentives can be tied to measures of clinical quality (often HEDIS measures), structural capacity (e.g., health IT), efficiency, or patient experience.

In the Medicare program, several significant PFP incentive programs have been incorporated into physician payments in the past decade as part of a broader initiative to increase the application of value-based payment in Medicare (CMS, undated [b]). Medicare's PFP incentives for physicians include bonuses for meaningful use of health IT and, more recently, incentive payments based on measures of clinical quality and efficiency (Fenter and Lewis, 2008; Hsiao et al., 2011). In 2007, CMS established a voluntary "pay-for-reporting" program in Medicare called the Physician Quality Reporting System (PQRS) under which an eligible physician could earn up to a 1.5-percent bonus applied to his or her Medicare rates based on quality measures (CMS, 2007). The PQRS program was made permanent in 2008, and incentive payments were authorized through 2010. Pursuant to the ACA, PQRS incentives were increased and extended through 2014, and CMS is now in the process of phasing in a mandatory PFP for all physicians under a program now called the Physician Value-Based Payment Modifier (PVBPM) (CMS, 2014a).

The PVBPM includes measures of clinical quality (e.g., eye exams for diabetics), as well as measures of efficiency based on the total costs of care, including nonphysician services. Measurement of quality and costs under the PVBPM started in 2013. Payments will be adjusted beginning in 2015 for physicians in large groups (100 or more) and, beginning in 2017, for all other physicians (Ryan and Damberg, 2013). Although Medicare payment rates will be adjusted by only a few percentage points under the PVBPM, it is significant for several reasons: The program is mandatory; it includes both bonuses and penalties; Medicare is the largest payer in the United States; and private health plans often model their physician payments on Medicare. Given physician payment legislation that Congress considered recently, there appears to be an intent to expand the application of PFP to Medicare physician payments (Elmendorf, 2014).

Outside the Medicare program, PFP is likely to be quite common, although its prevalence is difficult to gauge because there is no ongoing, systematic collection of data on physician payment models. From the CTS, we know that the use of PFP by commercial plans expanded in the mid-2000s and that, by 2005, health plans in all 12 of the CTS communities had implemented, or were planning to implement, some form of PFP (Trude, Au, and Christianson, 2006). And in a 2007–2009 survey of small and medium-sized physician practices, 61 percent "reported participating in a pay-for-performance or public reporting program" (Hearld et al.,

2014, p. 303). Among large medical groups responding to a telephone survey in 2006–2007, just over half reported that they "had received any additional income in the past year from health insurance plans based on clinical quality or patient satisfaction" (Robinson, Shortell, Rittenhouse, et al., 2009, p. 173).

The prevalence of PFP varies geographically and by type of health plan. PFP is ubiquitous in certain states, including California (Cromwell et al., 2011; Ryan and Damberg, 2013) and Massachusetts, where 89 percent of the leaders of primary care physician groups reported PFP incentives in at least one commercial health plan contract (Mehrotra et al., 2007). California has historically been "ahead of the curve" in the prevalence of alternative payment models (Zuvekas and Cohen, 2010); for the past decade, IHA has spearheaded payment reform efforts in that state (IHA, 2014). PFP also appears to be more commonly applied by HMO plans (Tisnado et al., 2008) and in payments to physicians participating in larger systems, such as IPAs, physician–hospital organizations (PHOs), or integrated delivery systems (Hearld et al., 2014). This is likely due to easier attribution of enrollees to physician practices and the prevalence of fully insured plans rather than self-insured plans. Not surprisingly, participation in voluntary PFP programs has been shown to be strongly and positively associated with the amount of the available incentives (de Brantes and D'Andrea, 2009).

Effects of Pay for Performance: Incentives and Interventions to Affect Individual Physician Decisionmaking

PFP incentives appear to "flow downhill," meaning that measuring health plan quality supports the application of PFP in payments to physician organizations, which, in turn, makes it more likely that individual physicians' compensation arrangements will include quality-based incentive payments (Robinson, Shortell, Rittenhouse, et al., 2009; Merritt Hawkins, undated; Merritt Hawkins, 2013). There is convincing evidence to show that PFP incentives can refocus physician practices' clinical activities and documentation and increase measured compliance with clinical guidelines (Chaix-Couturier et al., 2000). For example, an evaluation of a program offering $100 to patients and obstetricians or midwives for timely and comprehensive prenatal care found that adherence on 40 clinical process measures increased sharply (Rosenthal, Li, et al., 2009). An analysis of the rollout of IHA's California statewide PFP initiative in the mid-2000s found significant increases in several process measures (Rodriguez et al., 2009). One review found fairly consistent evidence that PFP incentives were associated with improved measures of processes of care (Petersen et al., 2006), and another recent review finds that, "[i]n general there was about 5% improvement [in clinical effectiveness] due to PFP use, but with a lot of variation, depending on the measure and program" (Van Herck et al., 2010, p. 4). And medical groups facing HEDIS-based PFP incentives are more likely to have in place ongoing quality improvement (QI) initiatives targeting those specific HEDIS measures (Mehrotra et al., 2007). Yet another recent review finds

> improvement in selected quality measures in most [PFP] initiatives, but the contribution of financial incentives to that improvement is not clear; the incentives typically were implemented in conjunction with other quality improvement efforts, or there was not a convincing comparison group. (Christianson, Leatherman, and Sutherland, 2008, p. 5S)

PFP's impact on physician practices is dampened by the fact that different health plans apply a cacophony of performance metrics, particularly given the small financial amounts typically involved. For example, one incentive program offering a 5-percent bonus was dismissed as "laughable, it isn't even worth doing" (Carroll, 2007).

Achieving high performance scores affects practice revenues, but our literature review did not reveal any instances in which PFP payments had direct, substantial effects on physician practices' overall financial viability.

Effects of Pay for Performance: Changes in Practice Organization and Goals

PFP incentives clearly favor physician organizations that have the analytical and management capacity to measure and improve quality and the capital to invest in EHRs (Miller, 2010). Small and solo practices can succeed under PFP, but they face increasing difficulties in keeping up with the various incentive programs. PFP programs might have contributed to a shift away from small and solo practices toward larger practices, but our search did not yield any previously published evidence indicating that participation in PFP had changed the way practices are organized.

One review of the evidence on PFP documented several cases of unintended consequences, including practices avoiding the sickest patients because of a belief that treating them would result in lower measured performance, and illusory improvements in quality that merely reflect improved documentation (Petersen et al., 2006). One serious criticism of PFP models is that current quality measures capture only a few very narrow slices of the range of a physician's activities (Berenson and Kaye, 2013). This has fostered concerns among some physicians that their attention is being diverted from "unincentivized" services and from broader self-directed quality goals (Eijkenaar et al., 2013).

Effects of Pay for Performance: Changes in Production Model for Patient Care

PFP increases administrative burden and reporting requirements, particularly for smaller practices and practices serving patients from many different health plans (Halladay et al., 2009). The administrative burden has been cited anecdotally as "a major reason for rising practice expenses" (Goldsmith, 2012, p. 57), although, according to survey responses, the reporting burden from multiple programs does not appear to be severe (Hearld et al., 2014). We did not uncover studies that quantified the level or types of staff or capital investments required to meet PFP requirements.

One study found that medical groups facing PFP incentives that promote the use of EHRs are significantly more likely than other groups to have adopted EHRs (Robinson, Casalino, et al., 2009). The requirements that practices collect and submit other quality measures could also indirectly encourage use of EHRs, although we did not identify any empirical studies investigating this mechanism of encouragement.

Effects of Pay for Performance: Physician Outcomes

We did not identify clear evidence of PFP's effect on the overall quantity of physician work, but a substantial literature addressed the effects that PFP programs have on physician motivation and satisfaction. Those effects appear to depend on the specifics of the program and the individual physician. Anecdotal reports cite the potential for significant increases in physician satisfaction following implementation of a well-designed and inclusive PFP program (Suarez, Byrne, and Bottles, 2003). Physicians in focus groups and surveys generally agree that PFP programs have the potential to motivate positive behavior change (Murphy and Nash, 2008), but they also "expressed significant anger about and suspicion of financial incentives for quality. Many viewed the incentive dollars as money already owed (i.e., 'a take-away and give-back masquerading as a bonus')" (Teleki et al., 2006, p. 371). Physicians whose compensation includes productivity bonuses were more likely than other physicians to express job dissatisfaction, but that relationship could reflect a tangled mix of other factors rather than the bonus arrangements per se (Grembowski et al., 2003).

When surveyed regarding a specific PFP program, medical directors of academic training programs expressed widespread skepticism regarding the accuracy of the performance measure and whether attaching financial incentives would improve care (Pines et al., 2007). And, in a survey of primary care physicians, 30 percent reportedly "viewed extrinsic pressures to standardize care as contrary to their clinical judgment," and that perception was associated with a higher likelihood of job dissatisfaction (Waddimba et al., 2013, p. 287).

Serious objections to PFP have been raised, on both conceptual and practical grounds. There is evidence that physicians' behavior is strongly driven by intrinsic motivation, i.e., the desire to perform well (including providing patient care they consider to be of high quality) irrespective of financial rewards (Friedberg, Chen, et al., 2013; Kolstad, 2013). In the context of such intrinsic motivation, tying financial incentives to quality of care could undermine physicians' professionalism (Beckman et al., 2006), lead physicians to "teach to the test" (Berenson, Pronovost, and Krumholz, 2013), and promote disproportionate or even excessive treatment of conditions, such as diabetes, with readily quantifiable clinical markers (Damberg et al., 2014). In a survey assessing physicians' views of different health plans, "physicians reported that the use of education and peer influence influenced their clinical behavior and facilitated the provision of high-quality care more than did rules and regulations or financial incentives" (Williams, Zaslavsky, and Cleary, 1999, p. 589).

Shared Savings Programs
Prevalence
The evidence in the existing literature regarding shared savings programs comes entirely from studies of ACOs. Therefore, in this section, all studies cited were conducted in ACOs, although we emphasize that ACOs combine elements of a variety of different payment models, including PFP and shared savings.

ACOs are a relatively recent innovation that has expanded very rapidly. CMS conducted some of the early experiments with ACOs (though the term had not been invented then) through the Medicare Physician Group Practice (PGP) Demonstration, which began in 2005 (CMS, 2011). PGP allowed group practices to share cost savings with Medicare as long as they met targets for quality of care, and it included ten multispecialty physician groups, each with at least 200 physicians, in ten states (Cromwell et al., 2011). CMS also began conducting the Physician–Hospital Collaboration Demonstration in 2009, which offers "gain-sharing" for physicians and hospitals.

In 2010, the ACA established ACOs as a national voluntary program supported by CMS for Medicare patients. In January 2013, more than 4 million beneficiaries received care in Medicare ACOs, equivalent to 11 percent of total Medicare FFS beneficiaries (Oliver Wyman, 2013), and CMS has reported that the number of Medicare beneficiaries in ACOs will rise to more than 7 million in 2015 (Cavanaugh, 2014). Private-sector ACOs—or similar arrangements with different names—have emerged as well, and the total number of Medicare and non-Medicare patients served by an organization with ACO arrangements amounted to between 37 million and 43 million, or roughly 14 percent of the population, in early 2013 (Oliver Wyman, 2013). The potential reach of ACOs can be extended to even a larger population; 227 ACOs were identified in mid-2012, with 55 percent of the U.S. population residing in areas with at least one ACO (V. Lewis, Colla, Carluzzo, et al., 2013).

Many shared savings arrangements between commercial health plans and providers that are similar to ACOs have emerged in the past few years. For example, several provider organizations in Massachusetts entered the Blue Cross Blue Shield Alternative Quality Contract in 2009 and 2010. Like Medicare ACOs, this program features shared savings contingent on achieving certain quality benchmarks (Chernew et al., 2011; Song et al., 2012), and the state also enacted a sweeping reform in 2012, Chapter 224, that "encourages the adoption and use of alternative payment methods" (Center for Health Information and Analysis, 2013, p. 1). As of December 2014, Leavitt Partners counted 672 ACOs in the United States (Leavitt Partners Accountable Care Cooperative, 2014). Overall estimates of the prevalence of shared savings programs, including those promulgated by payers other than CMS, are likely to vary because of differences in ACO definitions and counting methods.

Medicare ACO formation is associated with certain regional characteristics: In 2012, the share of FFS beneficiaries in ACOs was greater in the Northeast (11 percent) and Midwest (9 percent) than in the South (4 percent) and West (7 percent), but many are also joining from the South (Auerbach et al., 2013; V. Lewis, Colla, Carluzzo, et al., 2013). Areas with more ACOs tend to have higher percentages of hospital revenue from capitation or risk-sharing contracts, and all Medicare, Medicaid, and commercial ACOs were likely to form in areas with greater managed care penetration (Auerbach et al., 2013; V. Lewis, Colla, Carluzzo, et al., 2013). Some argue that ACOs are more likely to have formed in places where achievement is easier (i.e., costs are high and performance on quality measures is already superior; providers in that type of environment might be more confident about cutting costs and meeting quality standards) (V. Lewis, Colla, Carluzzo, et al., 2013).

At the end of the first year of Medicare's Pioneer ACO program (an ACO program designed for relatively large and experienced organizations with highly developed QI capabilities), most of the participating organizations scored higher on the quality targets than a Medicare FFS comparison group (Pham, Cohen, and Conway, 2014). However, since program inception, nine Pioneer ACOs have switched to the Medicare Shared Savings Program, and three Pioneer ACOs have dropped out without entering another Medicare ACO program. Some Pioneer organizations have reported that the number of performance measures used by the program was a significant burden, and measures not based on claims data have been costly to measure and submit to CMS (Hackbarth, 2014). Some participants reported challenges because of inadequate adjustment for patient disease severity and socioeconomic status, significant operating expense, and "leakage" where patients use non-ACO providers and incur unnecessary services (K. Patel and Lieberman, 2013).

The buzz around Medicare ACOs has spurred interest in commercial ACO contracting arrangements. In general, commercial ACO efforts are similar to those of Medicare ACO programs in shying away from limiting provider choice and self-referrals, requiring providers to meet various quality standards before sharing in savings, and focusing provider incentives on improving clinical performance rather than managing actuarial risk (Grossman, Tu, and Cross, 2013). There might also be some important differences, as indicated by a recent analysis of the National Survey of Accountable Care Organizations, which found that commercial (private health plan) ACO contracts were more likely than public-payer ACOs to include downside risks and up-front payments (e.g., for care management of capital investments) (V. Lewis, Colla, Schpero, et al., 2014).

In addition, state Medicaid agencies, plans, and providers are beginning to participate in innovative initiatives for their beneficiaries (McGinnis and Small, 2012). By mid-2013, at least nine states—Arkansas, Colorado, Illinois, Iowa, Minnesota, New Jersey, Oregon, Utah, and Vermont—had approved and adopted an accountable care model (Kocot et al., 2013). Unlike Medicare or commercial ACOs, Medicaid ACOs must weave financing and delivery for medical and social services at the community level, given their complex and vulnerable beneficiary population (McGinnis and Small, 2012). Although ample opportunities for coordination and cost reduction in Medicaid exist, especially for the dual-eligible population, challenges, such as assessing and distributing shared savings in the midst of federal–state financing arrangements, also exist (Kocot et al., 2013).

Different practice arrangements of ACO formation are possible: integrated or organized delivery system, multispecialty group practices, PHOs, IPAs, and "virtual" physician organizations (Shortell and Casalino, 2010). All five types suggest consolidation between similar and different types of providers. Empirically, Medicare ACOs are more likely to form in areas with high proportions of hospitals affiliated with integrated delivery systems (Auerbach et al., 2013), and larger practices and those with more-extensive care management processes were more likely to have joined ACOs (Shortell, McClellan, et al., 2014).

A large majority (60 percent) of the sample of physician practices in the NSPO in 2012 and 2013 reported no involvement and no plans to become involved in ACOs. Still, in the same survey, 24 percent reported joining ACOs, and 16 percent were planning to join (Shortell, McClellan, et al., 2014).

Effects of Shared Savings Programs: Incentives and Interventions to Affect Individual Physician Decisionmaking

There are anecdotal reports of ACOs implementing real-time feedback systems, and financial rewards, to improve care coordination and outcomes. For example, in one of the Pioneer ACOs, Banner Health Network,

> Population management software continually stratifies risk for the 50,000 beneficiaries in the ACO. Primary care physicians are notified about the high-risk outliers in their panel and prompted to ask those patients a predetermined set of questions designed to figure out why, say, they are going to the emergency department so often. Once physicians have entered the answers to those questions into the ACO's software—a case manager checks to make sure the answers are complete—they are rewarded $100 for referring the high-risk patient for a comprehensive action plan. (Wehrwein, 2013)

That type of ability to "push" information to physicians has been identified, in industry publications, as a key to ACOs performing successfully (Sandlot Solutions, 2012)—although, to our knowledge, no research studies have verified this claim.

In addition, an evaluation of the Medicare PGP demonstration suggested that physicians in participating groups intensified or increased the completeness of their diagnostic coding, a behavior change that would result in favorable shared savings calculations under the demonstration's concurrent risk-adjustment model (Kautter et al., 2012). Whether and how participating physician groups intervened with their physicians to change diagnostic coding practices was unclear.

Effects of Shared Savings Programs: Organizational Changes

The effects of ACOs are visible in the changes physicians make in their behavior and in their changing relationships with health plans and hospitals to achieve shared savings. For example, physicians are increasingly taking on significant leadership roles in ACOs. In the National Survey of ACOs from October 2012 to May 2013, 51 percent of the respondent ACOs reported being physician-led, 33 percent jointly led with a hospital, and 3 percent hospital-led. Respondents in physician-led ACOs expressed the most optimism about the ACO model's dissemination and potential to improve quality (V. Lewis, Colla, Carluzzo, et al., 2013). In addition, although four pilot ACOs from the Brookings–Dartmouth Collaborative varied in size, from 7,000 to 50,000 attributed patients and 90 to 2,700 participating physicians, all created shared savings agreements linked to quality measures by forming new, collaborative relationships with health plans (Larson et al., 2012). Others have reported that the process of implementing ACOs has required health plans to invest in developing provider capabilities, data sharing systems, and joint strategic planning with providers (Higgins et al., 2011; Claffey et al., 2012; Larson et al., 2012). Recent data also indicate that organizations with commercial ACO contracts are more complex (e.g., they were significantly more likely to be integrated delivery systems, have more providers, and include a hospital) than those with public ACO contracts only (V. Lewis, Colla, Schpero, et al., 2014).

Likewise, participants in Medicare's PGP program employed a range of strategies to improve quality and reduce cost, including coordinating care transitions, practicing evidence-based medicine, and coordinating and managing chronic and high-risk patients. Most participants were able to utilize existing IT and management infrastructure to respond to the new requirements and incentives (Kautter et al., 2012).

As ACOs encourage collaboration and accountability among providers, subsequent hospital mergers and provider consolidation could lead to greater integration among provider groups that wield market power in negotiations, forcing private insurers to pay more and driving up overall health care costs (Gaynor and Town, 2012). Even in the absence of integration, partners that come together to form a Medicare or Medicaid ACO have the potential to negotiate jointly with private payers, whether for an ACO contract or under FFS. In response, some have argued that consolidations are already a pervasive trend, with or without ACOs (Gold, 2011).

Effects of Shared Savings Programs: Physician Outcomes

Along with hopes that ACOs will transform care delivery and result in controlled costs, increased quality, and improved population health, skepticism toward the new model also abounds. Some have pointed out that ACOs heavily resemble the failed integrated delivery networks of the 1990s in their promises and that ample challenges still exist, such as substantial investment of money and time, lack of foreknowledge about which capabilities (e.g., care coordination, disease management) are necessary for success, and potential need for hiring new personnel, such as care coordinators and IT staff (Burns and Pauly, 2012). Participating providers are to be mindful of overestimating their organizational capabilities or their ability to manage risk and report performance measures (Singer and Shortell, 2011).

We did not discover any studies that directly assessed the effects that participation in an ACO has on physician professional satisfaction. Shields and his colleagues have suggested, though, that the opportunity to take a lead role in patient care without the daily interactions with managed care organizations is likely to be an incentive for joining (Shields et al., 2011).

Retainer and Concierge Payment Models

Although concierge care has received significant media attention recently, it has not been widely studied and appears to be a relatively uncommon, but growing, phenomenon. Estimates of the size of the concierge medicine market vary greatly. A 2013 article reported that fewer than 5,000 physicians have full concierge practices, meaning they accept annual membership fees for patient care and do accept health insurance, whereas a 2014 article stated that 100,000 patients are enrolled in more than 12,000 practices nationwide (Page, 2013; Frank, 2014). The key study, published in 2005, examining practice characteristics of retainer physicians is the Alexander et al. cross-sectional study of 83 retainer physicians and 231 nonretainer physicians (Alexander, Kurlander, and Wynia, 2005). The study found that most retainer practices were formed recently, with a mean of 17 months in practice, and most specialized in general internal medicine or family practice.

Lucier et al. reported on the academic retainer practice model, which was a collaboration between the Department of Medicine at Tufts University Medical Center and MDVIP, a concierge medicine company (Lucier et al., 2010). The goal of the program was not to exclude patients with limited ability to pay, but rather to cross-subsidize poorly reimbursed services. In this program, each physician retains no more than 275 retainer patients, along with approximately 900 patients from the general medical center. Each patient pays a yearly retainer fee of $1,800 in addition to charges for regular office visits.

Effects of Retainer and Concierge Models: Incentives and Interventions to Affect Individual Physician Decisionmaking

We found little published literature describing financial incentives or other interventions targeting individual physicians in retainer or concierge practices. A recent paper describing physician payment in ten health systems found that One Medical, a retainer-based primary care practice, paid its physicians on salary, with small adjustments for performance on measures of quality, service, and teamwork (Khullar et al., 2014).

Effects of Retainer and Concierge Models: Organizational Changes

Smaller patient panels are one of the key perceived advantages of concierge care, for both the physician and the patient. Alexander et al. found that panels for retainer physicians were less than half as large as nonretainer physicians (mean 898 versus 2,303; $p < 0.0001$). Although one of the perceived benefits is the ability to avoid interactions with health plans, the majority of retainer practices continue to accept payments from third-party insurers, either to satisfy patients who need to maintain their insurance in any case and would like to make use of its physician benefits or as a precaution in case they decide to abandon this model in the future (Page, 2013).

There was no evidence in the literature that retainer and concierge models are prompting practices to grow in size or consider new ownership models. We also did not identify any evidence of consistent changes in labor or capital needs in the practice, resulting from participation in retainer or concierge models.

Effects of Retainer and Concierge Models: Physician Outcomes

A strong contributing factor to the growth of concierge medicine is maintaining or increasing income while reducing patient panel size. Whereas average annual fees run $1,400 to $1,700, some practices charge as much as $25,000 (Bellafante, 2013). Although data on salaries are scant, trade press has reported that average salary ranges in retainer practices seem to largely overlap those in conventional practices (Horowitz, 2013).

Becoming a retainer practice introduces an organizational challenge, which is how to deal with patients who choose not to pay the new fee. Almost half (42 percent) of retainer physicians were highly involved with transferring care for patients who were not switching to the retainer practice, and two-thirds gave their patients at least three months to find a new provider.

Although evidence is anecdotal, it appears that the overall quantity and content of physician work is significantly altered by retainer and concierge payment, given the drastic reduction in patient panels, but we did not find peer-reviewed research evidence of these effects.

Medical Home Programs
Prevalence

Medical homes (or patient-centered medical homes) are a set of related primary care–focused health care–delivery models that have proliferated rapidly in the past several years. In the private sector, key organizations, such as NCQA, the Utilization Review Accreditation Committee, and the Joint Commission (Burton, Devers, and Berenson, 2012), and some commercial health plans, such as Blue Cross Blue Shield of Michigan, have developed and promoted standards for accrediting medical homes (Paustian et al., 2014). In the public sector, numerous agencies, including AHRQ, CMS, U.S. Department of Defense, Health Resources and Services Administration (HSRA), Substance Abuse and Mental Health Services Administration, and Veterans Health Administration, have been involved in further developing medical homes. Federal initiatives include funding for demonstrations, technical assistance, evaluation of current programs, and training programs. Under a medical home payment model, as a condition of contracting, health plans typically require physician practices to either be certified as medical homes or provide pay-for-structure incentives to such certified practices.

Five years ago, relatively few physician practices met the criteria to qualify as medical homes, and participation in medical home payment programs was rare. Analysis of the 2008 HTPS revealed that, at that time, approximately 41 percent of primary care physicians were in practices with minimal or no medical home services, and only 13.5 percent were in practices offering all of the "must-pass" medical home elements; solo and two-physician practices were even less likely to offer those elements (Ullrich, MacKinney, and Mueller, 2013). In 2009, the Patient-Centered Primary Care Collaborative cataloged 27 private-sector medical home pilot and demonstration projects (Patient-Centered Primary Care Collaborative, 2009). Also in 2009, a separate team of researchers found that 14,000 physicians were participating in a medical home pilot, caring for around 5 million patients (Bitton, Martin, and Landon, 2010). Since 2009, the number of practices involved in medical home initiatives has increased sharply (Edwards, Bitton, et al., 2014), rising to nearly 7,000 practices and 35,000 clinicians in 37 states in 2013 using NCQA standards and recognition (O'Kane, 2007). Blue Cross and Blue Shield plans have a parallel set of medical home programs running in 40 states and the District of Columbia serving more than 5 million members (Center for Health Information and Analysis, 2013), and the federal government, through Medicare, Medicaid, and other agencies, also has initiated multiple medical home demonstrations (AHRQ, undated).

Effects of Medical Home Programs: Incentives and Interventions to Affect Individual Physician Decisionmaking

We found little published evidence on incentives and interventions targeting individual physicians within medical homes. In particular, the degree and manner in which the enhanced payments commonly included in medical home pilots (e.g., care management fees) are distributed to physicians is unknown and might vary from practice to practice. However, anecdotal evidence suggests that some medical homes have taken steps to reduce the degree to which physician compensation is determined by RVU-based measures of utilization, a change that is consistent with the "comprehensive payment for comprehensive care" vision underlying some medical home models (Goroll et al., 2007). For example, in a qualitative study of five practices participating in a medical home pilot, physicians were paid salaries with bonuses (up to 25 percent of base salary) for performance on measures of quality, efficiency, and patient experience of care (Bitton, Schwartz, et al., 2012). Similarly, in a medical home intervention conducted within the Seattle-based Group Health Cooperative, physician salaries were delinked from RVU-based measures of productivity, a change intended to incentivize performance of non–visit-based care (Reid et al., 2009).

Effects of Medical Home Programs: Changes in Organization and Production Model for Patient Care

Larger physician practices tend to be better prepared to participate in medical home initiatives (Rittenhouse, Casalino, Gillies, et al., 2008; Friedberg, Safran, et al., 2009; Rittenhouse, Casalino, Shortell, et al., 2011) and might have greater capacity for change (Hearld et al., 2014). Medical home designation might require investment in IT, extensive documentation, and payment of a recognition fee, all of which could limit participation by smaller practices that lack the resources to invest in the requisite medical home infrastructure. It is unclear, however, whether the proliferation of medical home initiatives has prompted physicians in solo practice or very small groups to join larger practices.

Medical home practices have been found to have significantly higher-than-average ratios of support-staff full-time equivalents to physician full-time equivalents (M. Patel et al., 2013). In terms of the roles of administrative and clinical support staff, medical home–designated primary care practices are more likely to employ care managers or coordinators but are otherwise generally similar to other primary care practices (Peikes et al., 2014).

Medical home programs promote greater interactions and tighter relationships between physician practices and their parent physician organizations (Wise et al., 2012) and commonly involve some type of learning collaborative designed to assist practices in their QI efforts (Bitton, Martin, and Landon, 2010; Edwards, Bitton, et al., 2014). A 2012 qualitative study of five practices initiating medical home programs found that, by seeking out efficiencies through either population health management or driving out waste, nurses and other health professional were able work closer to the top of their licenses, more staff could be hired, and physicians were able to either accept new patients or spend more time with complex cases. Teamwork was increased by each practice via daily meetings, checklists, or regular feedback (Bitton, Schwartz, et al., 2012). A qualitative study of a national sample of NCQA-recognized medical homes found that teamwork in medical homes featured expanded roles for medical assistants (MAs) and nurses, facilitated by template-guided data-gathering and previsit planning "huddles" between physicians and other practice staff, as well as prominent roles for nurse care managers (O'Malley, Gourevitch, et al., 2015).

Effects of Medical Home Programs: Physician Outcomes

Cross-sectional analyses have suggested that practices exhibiting medical home characteristics tend to have higher staff morale (S. Lewis et al., 2012) and lower rates of burnout (K. Nelson et al., 2014), although longitudinal evaluations that measure the effects of medical home implementation are lacking, limiting our knowledge of whether and which medical home implementations actually improve morale (Friedberg, 2012). On a cautionary note, one longitudinal study in the Veterans Health Administration showed that physician turnover actually increased following medical home implementation, suggesting that some physicians had negative experiences (Sylling et al., 2014).

Semistructured interviews with 12 primary care teams with the highest Medical Home Index scores in a national medical home initiative identified four essential medical home attributes as drivers of transformation: (1) a culture of QI, (2) family-centered care with parents as improvement partners, (3) team-based care, and (4) care coordination (McAllister et al., 2013).

One study surveying primary care teams participating in a national medical home initiative observed increased satisfaction among participating physicians and coordinators. However, clinicians were critical of the lack of support and strains of QI. Concerns included inequitable risks from caring for complex patients, sustaining their mission while adjusting to standards that demanded an unsupported level of quality, the pediatric medical home being neglected in the face of chronically ill adults, and that medical home activities becoming overwhelming and requiring personal time during evenings and weekends (McAllister et al., 2013). As the prevalence of medical home programs increases, participants will need to carefully plan and provide sufficient support in order for the desired changes to be realized.

Our literature review did not identify published research that evaluated the effects that participation in medical home programs has on the quantity of physician work or overall physician compensation.

CHAPTER FOUR

Methods

Overview of Methodological Approach

To describe the effects that payment models have on physician practices, this project employed qualitative methods, incorporating multiple case studies, with each of 34 physician practices constituting a case (Yin, 2014). Because the project sought to incorporate contextual information on market-level characteristics that might affect how practices respond to alternative payment models (e.g., the mix of competitors, health plans, and payment programs operating in the geographic area served by each practice), these 34 cases were nested within six geographically defined health care markets in the United States. We included a relatively large total number of cases because we sought to capture a diversity of practice sizes, specialties, and ownership models within each of six markets—a positivist approach allowing assessment of whether findings replicated across cases and offering a degree of generalizability (Yin, 2014). Thus, for each market, we gathered data from physician practices and other market participants and observers: leaders of health plans and hospitals operating in the market, state or county medical societies, and state Medical Group Management Association (MGMA) chapters.

The goal of this project was to identify a variety of practice models that are likely to enable successful long-term implementation of reform and to present actionable study findings, tailored to physician practices at different stages of integration and readiness for change. Given these goals, we chose physician practices as the primary unit of observation, but, when practices were nested within larger organizations, such as IPAs, we also sought to gather data from leadership the larger organization.

Justification for Qualitative Methods

The effects of new payment programs (alone and in combination) on physicians' professional activities and physician practices are largely unknown, and we did not have an existing taxonomy of these effects. Therefore, we chose a qualitative case-study design, which allowed us to detect, explore in depth, and categorize experiences of physicians and physician practices that we did not necessarily anticipate.

The design of the project was iterative, with periodic input on data collection methods and interpretation of results from members of the research team and the project advisory committee. Important changes were made throughout the project, particularly in its early stages, rather than fixed in advance. Specifically, we added to and refined the interview guides for physician practices based on findings from interviews with market observers (leaders of health plans, hospitals, medical societies, and MGMA chapters). The majority of these market-observer interviews occurred before the first interviews with physicians and physician practice leaders. Similarly, we modified our conceptual model based on emerging qualitative themes and used this model to generate additional interview questions, to guide qualitative codebook development, and to organize our findings.

Data Collection

Overview

Between April and November 2014, the project gathered data from 81 interviewees among 34 physician practices in six markets throughout the country: Little Rock, Arkansas; Orange County, California; Miami, Florida; Boston, Massachusetts; Lansing, Michigan; and Greenville, South Carolina. In addition, in order to examine market-context factors influencing the adoption of payment models and their implementation in practices, we also collected data from leaders of ten health plans, nine hospitals and hospital systems, seven medical societies, and five MGMA chapters (31 market-context interviews total).

The RAND Human Subjects Protection Committee approved all components of this research project. Participants in all data collection activities gave informed consent to participate in this research.

Market Selection

We selected six geographic markets from the 12 communities included in the CTS and HTPS. There were two advantages to this approach. First, the community reports from each CTS round contained information that could be used to help select markets and identify potential interviewees in each. Second, we reasoned that physician practices and other stakeholders in these markets might be accustomed to responding to requests from researchers for site visits and other data collection efforts.

In Table 4.1, we present the six markets, which we selected based on information from the most recent CTS community reports to maximize diversity on market context (provider market concentration, payer market concentration, and hospital roles) and payment models (prevalent in 2010 and likely changes since 2010).

Market Context: Sample of Interviewees

In each market, we invited interviewees in each of the following categories to participate in semistructured interviews that focused on the following content areas:

- *leaders of state and county medical societies and MGMA chapters:* These interviews gathered information on the history of the market and the evolution of physician practices within it. These interviews also served as an important source of suggestions for health plans and hospitals in the market for inclusion in the study.
- *leaders of health plans with significant market share:* These interviews gathered information on payment models used by each plan, changes and reasons for changes to these models, and suggestions for physician practices and hospitals to include in the study.
- *leaders of hospitals with significant market share:* These interviews gathered information on payment models in which each hospital participates, changes in these models, and past,

Table 4.1
Study Market Characteristics

Market	Market Context			Payment Model	
	Provider Characteristics	Payer Characteristics	Hospital Characteristics	Current in 2010	Trend in 2010
Boston, Massachusetts[a]	There is a high percentage of specialists. Outside of teaching hospitals, direct physician employment is rare, but alignment with hospitals is increasing.	There are three major commercial health plans—all regional—but the Blue Cross Blue Shield plan is much larger than others.	Academic hospital–based medical centers and one for-profit hospital chain dominate.	HMOs use capitation when contracting with large multispecialty groups. Substantial use of PFP in both HMOs and PPOs.	Alternative quality contract for HMO enrollees from Blue Cross Blue Shield consists of global payment with prominent PFP.
Greenville, South Carolina[b]	There are high levels of physician employment by hospitals. There are few independent physicians and no large independent multispecialty groups or IPAs.	Blue Cross Blue Shield has 60% of the commercial market.	There are two large and two small hospital systems with niche markets.	PPOs dominate, and there are high levels of patient cost-sharing.	There is much interest in ACOs given high rates of physician–hospital alignment.
Lansing, Michigan[c]	There are many small practices and few moderate or large groups. There is increasing physician employment by hospitals. Larger practices have achieved or are seeking medical home recognition.	Blue Cross Blue Shield has 70% of the commercial market, and an HMO subsidiary has an additional 10% of the market.	Two major hospital systems make up 90% of the market; the smaller of these hospital systems focuses on profitable specialty lines.	FFS is predominant.	The Blue Cross Blue Shield PFP program is well received by physicians as a means of supplementing low base payment rates. There is much interest in ACOs.
Miami, Florida[d]	Most physicians are in small independent primary care practices or specialty groups of fewer than 50 and admit to multiple hospitals.	The payer market is relatively unconcentrated with no dominant payer.	There are important nonprofit and for-profit systems, but none is dominant in the market as a whole. Hospitals are historically geographically segmented with little competition, but there is greater competition to attract wealthier patients.	There is a strong HMO market in both Medicare Advantage and commercial sectors.	Little payment innovation is occurring. Physician payment rates are very low overall. Cost containment focuses on lower-cost products with limited benefits.

Table 4.1—Continued

Market	Market Context			Payment Model	
	Provider Characteristics	Payer Characteristics	Hospital Characteristics	Current in 2010	Trend in 2010
Orange County, California[e]	Many physicians are in solo or small practices; physicians historically join multiple IPAs to contract for HMO patients. The number of IPAs each physician joins is decreasing.	There is no dominant payer. Anthem Blue Cross had 33% of the market, Kaiser 20%.	There is an unconsolidated hospital sector with three systems making up 50% of the market. There is growing interest in hospital–physician affiliations.	There is a high HMO share, in which the delegated model is widespread. FFS PPOs, including limited-benefit PPOs, and HMOs with deductibles are growing.	ACOs are anticipated to provide opportunity in the PPO and traditional Medicare space to use developed risk-management infrastructure to capture financial rewards for already-efficient care.
Little Rock, Arkansas[f]	Most physicians work in small, independent practices, with relatively few large multispecialty groups.	Blue Cross Blue Shield has nearly 70% of the commercial market, and two other plans divide the remainder.	There are three large hospital systems, all of which are statewide referral centers.	There is little experience with non-FFS payment models; most efforts to trim costs come through reductions in services and choice.	Medicaid expansion could present opportunity for experimentation with new payment models.

NOTE: PPO = preferred-provider organization.

[a] Tu, Dowling, et al., 2010.

[b] O'Malley, Anglin, et al., 2011.

[c] Tu, Anglin, et al., 2011.

[d] Christianson, Bond, et al., 2011.

[e] Felland et al., 2011.

[f] Christianson, Carrier, et al., 2011.

current, and anticipated relationships between the hospital and physician practices in the market.

To identify potential market-context interviewees, we used the most recent CTS reports for each market to identify the hospitals and health plans with the largest market shares. We then called each of these organizations, starting with the chief executive officer's (CEO's) office, to request a referral to the appropriate person within the organization's leadership. We identified the leaders of state and county medical societies by referral from the AMA, and similarly, we identified leaders of state MGMA chapters by referral from the national MGMA. We invited 45 potential market-context interviewees to participate in the study, and 31 consented to participate.

We asked each market-context interviewee to nominate physician practices for inclusion in the study (i.e., we used a snowball sampling strategy for physician practices). Neither physician membership in the AMA nor in the corresponding state medical society was required for potential inclusion. In seeking nominations, we specified our interest both in practices with a range of experiences in new payment programs, including those with varying lengths of experience with and successfulness in these payment programs (i.e., explicitly seeking to avoid creating a sample that included only those practices that were the earliest or most successful adopters of a given payment model).

Practice Sample

For the purpose of our study, a physician practice was defined as a business entity that accepted payment to support clinical care delivered by physicians. Such practices could range from solo practices to large corporations (with or without inclusion of hospitals or other facilities). Some practices had relationships with each other (e.g., through IPAs). As long as these practices were distinct businesses (each with its own balance sheet and ability to struggle or thrive financially on its own), we treated them as separate physician practices. However, we counted all sites of a given business entity (e.g., a large medical group with multiple locations) as a single physician practice.

Although some alternative payment models have focused historically on outpatient care delivered by primary care physicians, payment programs, such as shared savings, episode-based and bundled payments, and PFP, encompass or directly involve subspecialist physicians and hospitals. Therefore, we sought to include subspecialists and hospital-based practices in our data collection efforts.

Using nominations from the market-context interviews, we developed lists of practices in each market for potential inclusion in the study. After gathering initial information on each nominated practice's size, specialty, and ownership model, we invited selected practices to participate until six participants per market were identified, aiming for diversity on each of these practice design dimensions. This sampling design prioritized diversity of experience and did not attempt to generate a nationally representative sample of all physicians or physician practices in the United States.

We invited 89 physician practices to participate in the study, reminding each invited practice in a given market of our continued interest until we had recruited six practices in that market. To create a diverse sample of respondents within each market, we did not continue to recruit a given practice if another two practices in the same category (e.g., two other small, independent primary care practices) had consented to participate already. At the close of data collection, 34 physician practices consented to participate. Eleven invited physician practices explicitly declined to participate, most frequently citing competing time commitments as the reason for nonparticipation. Table 4.2 describes the sample of participating practices.

As shown in Table 4.2, we succeeded in achieving diversity on each practice design dimension. However, we were unable to sample practices with every *combination* of dimensions (as represented by the empty cells in Table 4.2). In some cases, these combinations are relatively rare (e.g., a large single-specialty practice or a small multispecialty practice).

Each practice could participate in multiple alternative payment models. Among these 34 physician practices, ten participated in global capitation, five in episode-based payments, 24 in PFP, 13 in shared savings (virtual global capitation), eight in medical home programs, and two in retainer or concierge payment models.

Data Collection: Semistructured Interviews

Prior to conducting the semistructured interviews, we developed interview guides for each type of respondent: medical society or MGMA chapter leader, health plan leader, hospital leader, physician practice leader, and practicing physician. As appropriate to semistructured interviews, interviewers followed respondents' leads, allowing the breadth and sequence of topics to flow naturally from respondents' answers to questions opening each topic. Each interview lasted 45 to 60 minutes. With respondent consent, we recorded and transcribed each interview.

To develop the interview guides, we drew on existing research and gray literature (reviewed in Chapter Three) to form an initial set of questions for each type of interviewee, based on early versions of our conceptual model. We refined the interview guides to facilitate better capture of themes emerging from early interviews. The final interview guides are available in Appendix B, available online.

Market-Context Interviews

We interviewed each of the market-context interviewees (health plan leaders, hospital leaders, and state and county medical society and MGMA chapter leaders) between April and August 2014. Interviews were conducted via phone by a team consisting of a physician interviewer and at least one note taker. In total, we conducted 31 such interviews: Leaders of ten health plans, nine hospitals and hospital systems, seven state or county medical societies, and five MGMA

Table 4.2
Physician Practice Sample

Practice Size	Physician-Owned or Partnership			Hospital or Corporate Owner		
	Multispecialty	Primary Care	Single Subspecialty[a]	Multispecialty	Primary Care	Single Subspecialty[a]
Large (>50 physicians)	4			4	2	
Medium (10–49 physicians)			4		1	2
Small (<9 physicians)		4	6	1	4	2

[a] Subspecialties represented include cardiology, gastroenterology, general surgery, neurology, obstetrics and gynecology, oncology, ophthalmology, orthopedic surgery, psychiatry, and vascular surgery.

chapters participated. Each market contained at least one respondent in each of the interviewee types (except MGMA chapter leaders, who were unable to participate in one market).

Physician Practices

We visited each of the 34 participating practices between August and November 2014. In each practice, we sought to interview the following types of respondents:

- practice leaders (not necessarily physicians; often professional managers), about payment models in which the practice participated and the effects of these payment models on practice growth, structural changes, financial position, and other aspects of the practice as an organization
- physicians who regularly deliver clinical care, about their professional experiences, including the quantity and content of work, care team structure and distribution of tasks, professional satisfaction, financial and nonfinancial incentives, and recent or anticipated changes in these aspects of clinical work.

For each practice that had multiple sites (e.g., large multispecialty practices), we visited one to four sites. To select these sites, we worked with practice leaders to identify a sample that would represent the typical range of physician experiences within the practice, including multiple specialties when possible.

One lead interviewer and at least one note taker conducted each interview. Most interviews were with individuals, but, to accommodate respondent schedules, some were with groups of interviewees. We performed the majority of interviews on site to facilitate rapport with interview subjects. We did not observe patient care directly. In total, we performed 81 semistructured interviews in physician practices (mean 2.4 per practice; range one to five): 26 with practice leaders who were not physicians, 22 with practice leaders who were physicians, and 33 interviews with practicing physicians who did not have leadership positions.

Data Collection: Practice Payment and Financial Position

To supplement the data collected in our interviews, we developed a practice financial questionnaire to be completed after interviews were conducted. The questionnaire asked about practice participation in alternative payment pilots or demonstrations, types of payers and payments received, and other financial measures on revenues, costs and expenditures, and income or loss. This questionnaire was adapted from existing surveys of practice finances, including the MGMA Cost Survey. For each practice visited, we asked the practice administrator, office manager, or other practice leader who seemed most knowledgeable about practice finances to fill out the questionnaire after the semistructured interviews was complete.

Data Analysis

An eight-person multidisciplinary team, including a general internist, a general pediatrician, and six policy researchers, each with training and expertise in qualitative methods and health services research, performed the qualitative analyses. Seven of the eight members of the data-analysis team also performed site visits and conducted the semistructured interviews and therefore were familiar with the data.

The team developed a code structure using systematic, inductive procedures to generate insights grounded in the views the study participants had expressed (Bradley, Curry, and Devers, 2007). To do this, the qualitative analysis team met weekly throughout the project to discuss each site visit, expand and refine a running list of key concepts identified from each interview, and draft and refine a conceptual model to organize and define relationships between identified concepts. The list of concepts, grouped into emerging categories, served as the initial codebook for qualitative analysis. Using this codebook, the team coded the interview transcripts, using the constant comparative method to ensure that themes were consistently classified, while allowing expansion of existing codes, identification of novel concepts, and refinement of codes (Bradley, Curry, and Devers, 2007). Following the multiple case-study framework (Yin, 2014), each interview with a practice leader or physician was coded in the context of the payment models in which the practice participated (which was a practice-level variable that did not vary within the practice).

The qualitative analysis team used essential components of consensual qualitative research to code the interview transcripts, including consensually agreeing on the meaning of the data and auditing the work of each qualitative coder to ensure consistency (Kvale, 1996; Hill et al., 2005). Specifically, each member of the coding team coded a set of interview transcripts independently. Two senior members of the coding team cross-checked each other's coding to ensure a common coding approach, then checked the work of the other coders. Any coder could suggest new codes for inclusion in the codebook; codebook additions or refinements were discussed by the qualitative analysis team and decided by consensus.

We used Dedoose version 4.5 (by SocioCultural Research Consultants in Los Angeles) to manage and analyze qualitative data.

Limitations

Our methods have limitations. First, because data collection required time commitments from practice leaders and physicians and did not offer financial compensation for their participation, severely struggling practices (i.e., those for which study participation would be a financial hardship) might have been underrepresented. Second, interview responses could have been subject to social-desirability bias, in which interviewees might have given answers that they felt would be more "socially acceptable" than their true beliefs. Our informed-consent checklist, which included an assurance of anonymity, was intended to help mitigate this source of bias. Third, our sampling plan was driven by practical considerations, such as the project timeline and available resources, rather than an explicit goal to reach theoretical saturation. Although it is possible that we did not reach theoretical saturation given these considerations, we do note that, toward the end of our data collection period, additional interviews were not reshaping our overall theory or conceptual model, indicating that theoretical saturation had likely been reached. Finally, our findings might not generalize to other markets or future time periods in which the payment programs that we investigated become more mature and physician practices become more familiar with them.

PART TWO

Results

The following chapters present the findings from our study. We note that this report has been written so that each chapter can be read and understood on its own, without having read earlier chapters.

CHAPTER FIVE

Changes in Organizational Structure

Overview of Findings

Multiple practice leaders and market-context interviewees reported that their own practices or others in their markets were changing their organizational models—predominantly by affiliating or merging with other physician practices or aligning with or becoming owned by hospitals—in response to new payment models.

From the physician practice perspective, the most prominent payment model–related reasons for these mergers were to enhance practices' ability to make the capital investments required to succeed in certain alternative payment models (especially investments in computers and data infrastructure), to negotiate contracts with health plans (including which performance measures and targets would be included), and to gain a sense of "safety in numbers." In addition, interviewees in multiple practices described uncertainty about how they would fare in new payment programs (and how such programs might evolve over time). For some of these practices, joining with a larger organization was seen as providing a general sense of security, no matter which payment programs might ultimately materialize.

The reported effects of alternative payment models on practice stability, including overall financial impact, ranged from neutral to positive. No practice in our sample indicated experiencing major financial hardship as a result of new payment models.

The retainer-based practices in our sample were small, and their physician-owners described their conversions to retainer-based payment as enabling an escape from market pressures that might otherwise have led to merger with other practices or early retirement.

Detailed Findings

Capital Investment Requirements Leading to Growth, Merger, and Hospital Affiliation or Ownership

The level of investment needed to participate successfully in many alternative payment models is not negligible and often requires a substantial amount of capital. A variety of practice respondents and market observers from across all study markets underlined the financial burden introduced by new payment models, often driven by the need to effectively manage payment models. The ability to manage effectively is often dependent on the ability to invest—in people, in technology, and in designing and implementing care processes.

A variety of practice respondents, most frequently those from small, physician-owned practices, reported that finding the capital to make vital investments in alternative payment models could be quite challenging. As one respondent summarized,

> Many of these small practices that are in rural areas, they're not going to go spend a ton of money to become a level 3 patient-centered medical home. They don't necessarily have that capital, and they're not necessarily in a situation where they can obtain it. In many cases, for some of these doctors out there, it's just not feasible to participate in an ACO or a patient-centered medical home if they're trying to practice independently and they're in a rural part of the state or an underserved location. . . . If they're really interested in participating in one of these models, then they might seek out an employment agreement, or . . . if it's a small practice and they're struggling to acquire the financial capital . . . can they merge?
>
> —leader, medical society

Similarly, some small, independent practices in particular noted that access to credit had become more difficult, increasing the attractiveness of hospitals and other large systems as sources of capital. In one market, even obtaining a modest line of credit had become more difficult after the recent financial crisis:

> There was a time . . . 15, 16, 17 years ago, where you walked into a bank . . . and they just literally said, "How much do you want?" and opened a business credit card line of $15,000, $30,000 immediately. . . . But it ran out; those times are over. [Tightening credit] started before the financial crisis . . . but then the financial crisis literally hammered it. The access to cheap credit was gone. . . . You can get access to money, but at very high interest rates now.
>
> —primary care physician, solo practice

As an alternative to relying on larger provider organizations (hospitals or large medical groups) to finance capital investment, one market observer suggested that health plans could serve this function directly, which could improve care for patients across multiple payers and insurance products:

> I think, for a lot of groups starting out, the health plans need to help them pay for the infrastructure that they have to build, and the health plans have to really [adopt] the mind-set that they don't have to help pay for the infrastructure forever, but, as a [physician practice] is beginning to [participate in risk-based payment], the health plans need to really help; and . . . if you look at groups that are successful in the risk business and the HMO world, they're also significantly less [costly in] the PPO world, because doctors tend to do the same thing and treat patients similarly, no matter what their insurance is.
>
> —leader, IPA participating in multiple shared savings and capitation programs

Physician Practices' Other Reasons for Growth, Merger, and Hospital Affiliation or Ownership

Better Negotiating Positions

Although no interviewee reported that enhancing a negotiating position was the sole reason for merging with other practices, becoming employed by hospitals, or affiliating with IPAs, physicians and practice leaders, particularly those in independent practices, noted that such organizational changes did improve their treatment by health plans. For example, one physician practice that had joined an IPA perceived that, as a group of physician practices, they were able to negotiate with payers more successfully:

> Because of the challenges in this state with the plans essentially being very aggressive in their contract negotiations . . . we developed our own IPA. . . . We have clinical committees, care management committees; we've really focused on not just the financial model, but the clinical model. . . . Our experience is that we've found more-favorable treatment in working through our IPA. And so as a result of that, that's how we were able to really negotiate the per-member per-months, by documenting the value of what we bring as a network and improved outcomes, lower cost, less emergency room utilization, so that was our leverage for negotiating.
>
> —administrative leader, large hospital-owned primary care practice

Another practice reported being empowered by being a relatively large group of specialists in a market faced with continued decline in FFS payment rates:

> From about the '90s when we had, as we called them, the bottom feeders who were willing to take anything . . . I think they were afraid. They thought they weren't ever going to be able to make a living if they didn't take what was offered to them. And doctors are not typically great negotiators. . . . They just want to see their patients. And so the 600-lb. gorilla would come into the room and say, "I'm only going to pay you this," and the guy would say, "Okay, all I want to do is go back in the exam room and see the next patient." And so that just ratcheted down the reimbursement, and it's particularly bad in [my specialty]. I think it's lack of cohesion. I think it's all these single practitioners who were out there who were afraid that they'd just get cut out and so they just said yes to anything and they allowed themselves to be bullied because they were individual practitioners. Part of the reason we came together as a group was so that we could have a united front.
>
> —administrator, medium-sized single-specialty practice

Perception of Greater Security in Changing and Unfamiliar Payment Models

Without citing specific payment models that led to a decision to affiliate with or become owned by a larger hospital or delivery system, some physicians and practice leaders described a sense of uncertainty concerning new payment models in general. This sentiment was expressed by a wide variety of respondents in all study markets, but most frequently by respondents from small, independent primary care practices. For these interviewees, joining forces with a large organization provided a sense of security—basically, that they would be harder to push around, no matter what new payment models lay in wait for them. Other market observers held similar views:

> There's a void of leadership out there for physicians and particularly the independent world; they're a little afraid. You know, they hear what's coming. They don't have the knowledge or expertise or capacity to address the issues that are coming. . . . When they see the amount of infrastructure and things that [hospital] can bring to the table and see the differences between even being part of a network as an independent doc versus being employed, they feel more secure being employed. And I think right now, security is probably outweighing their need for independence because the world is changing so quickly and they don't know how to address it otherwise.
>
> —leader, hospital

However, not all physician practices in our sample were interested in joining larger groups. Many respondents from small, independent practices perceived that joining larger systems would require them to give up more control and autonomy than they were willing to surrender. This was especially true for physician practices that were predominantly paid FFS or that could participate in new payment models (e.g., PFP programs) that did not require large patient populations or specific capital investments. As one respondent described,

> We were approached by a large multispecialty group to maybe join them. I actually kind of looked into that a little bit. Really didn't seem to be all that useful or valuable to us. . . . The pros were basically maintaining a stable referral base because it was a large multispecialty group. Everything else was kind of cons. Relinquishing some control over management, relinquishing control over contract negotiations, revenue disbursements, schedules.
>
> —physician, small physician-owned single-subspecialty practice

Effects on Practice Sustainability

Few respondents reported that alternative payment models had large effects on physician practices' financial stability (i.e., financial gains or losses sufficient to change a practice's ability to continue as a business). Some practice leaders attributed this lack of effect to the alternative payment models being implemented recently and accounting for a relatively modest share of their practices' total revenues. At the same time, such early and relatively low-stakes participation in alternative payment models was often viewed as a "dry run" for what was widely believed to be the future predominant model of payment. Although this was noted in most study markets, it was most commonly reported by medium-sized and large physician-owned primary care and multispecialty practices. For this respondent, a dry run was a way for a practice with little experience in taking risk to rehearse mechanisms for identifying desirable changes regardless of payment model:

> So the [shared savings program] as a payment model is probably not that material of a payment model from a financial perspective. That said, we are a very risk-averse organization, and we've also identified the [shared savings program] as kind of the first thing we wanted to get into with respect to risk, so it has had a disproportionate impact on folks. . . . If we didn't focus on it, we wouldn't lose our shirts; in fact, it would probably be a rounding

error. But it kind of stimulates the work; it gives us data, and it allows us to identify some of these opportunities.

—leader, large multispecialty practice

Similarly, the investments required to perform well in alternative payment models could counterbalance the additional payments received, resulting in little net effect on practice finances, especially when these additional payments lagged practices' investments. As one participant in a medical home pilot described,

So when we became [a medical home], we had invested in the practice. We hired two care managers and a little bit more staff. And of course that's expensive, and, when you're hiring more people and [you] already aren't making ends meet, it's just a loss. And so we needed some [financial] support for the medical home, [but] the payment for it has been very slow in coming. . . . I think more of our positive return is on kudos and recognition than it has been on money.

—physician, medium-sized primary care practice

Retainer Models Have Offered an Escape for Some Small Practices

In this study, all participating retainer practices were owned by solo practitioners, who were consistently pleased with their decisions to transition to retainer models of payment. Although these retainer practices continued to bill third-party payers, most frequently through FFS, the majority of practice revenue came from retainer fees. As a result of dramatically reducing dependency on third-party payment, these physicians reported feeling freer to practice medicine as they chose and avoiding financial pressure to join a larger organization or retire:

I reached a point where I was exhausted [and] financially I was having trouble paying my bills. [Other practices in the retainer model were] practicing the same way I was practicing. They were seeing their own patients in the hospital . . . returning all of their phone calls . . . working as solo practitioners . . . seeing 600 patients and making a living. . . . [After adopting the retainer model], all of a sudden, I had money coming in, no matter what the insurances were. Since I didn't have the same amount of patients . . . I had time. I didn't have to rush with my patients.

—physician-owner, solo retainer-based primary care practice

Comparison Between Current Findings and Previously Published Research

Our findings suggest that some alternative payment models might encourage practices to seek different models of organization, particularly by growing in size, merging with hospitals, or affiliating with larger organizations. These findings are concordant with previous research indicating that larger organizations might be better prepared for participation in PFP, shared savings, and medical homes. This could be due to better analytical and management capacity among larger organizations for measuring and improving quality (Miller, 2010). Other existing work has shown that larger physician practices might be better prepared to participate in medical home initiatives because they have more-advanced structural capabilities at baseline (Rittenhouse, Casalino, Gillies, et al., 2008; Friedberg, Safran, et al., 2009; Rittenhouse, Casalino, Shortell, et al., 2011) and greater capacity for change (Hearld et al., 2014). However, the direction of causality that might underlie observed associations in previous cross-sectional research is uncertain; it remains unclear whether the payment models are driving organizational change or whether organizations meeting certain criteria (e.g., larger size, greater resources to support data) are simply more likely to participate in certain payment models. Although the current study cannot prove that causal relationships exist, interviewees did perceive that certain requirements of alternative payment models (especially the need to make large investments in physician practices) are leading to greater consolidation.

CHAPTER SIX

Changes in Practice Operations

Overview of Findings

Respondents to our study perceived that alternative payment models have encouraged the development of team approaches to care management, featuring prominent roles for allied health professionals. In primary care practices in particular, physicians and practice leaders described appreciating how payment models, such as medical home and shared savings (based on virtual global capitation), had allowed them to fund care manager positions. These dedicated care managers, who were allied health professionals in all cases in our sample, could concentrate on patient management between office visits, alleviating some of the pressure that physicians would feel if these activities were added to already-packed visits.

Alternative payment models that incentivize containment of total costs of care also increased the importance of offering expanded options for patients to access care from physician practices. Two examples of such expanded access were communication options for after-hours care (via web portal or telephone) and provision of in-person care in the community, outside the office.

Because global capitation and related shared savings models focus predominantly on primary care services for patient attribution and performance measurement, market observers and physician practices reported that these alternative payment models were changing relationships between primary care physicians and subspecialist physicians. In some cases, these changes were collaborative, with multispecialty teams working to prevent progression of disease, without necessarily changing referral patterns. In other cases, changes in referral relationships were the main changes described because alternative payment models led practices to reduce "leakage" to subspecialists in other organizations.

Detailed Findings

Teamwork to Perform Care Management

Respondents in practices of all specialties and in all markets, with the exception of physicians in solo retainer-based practices, described how allied health professionals performed an expanded scope of tasks under alternative payment models. The role of allied health professionals was particularly prominent in performing care management, an activity often described as a "team sport." With teammates shouldering care management work in medical home, shared savings, and, to some extent, episode-based and bundled payment models, these activities could occur outside of already-packed physician office visits:

> Our general philosophy has been that you have to create the care management infrastructure to be able to support [physicians'] efforts. You can't expect the doc, in their 15- and 20-minute appointments, to do all this stuff. So you have to have the population manager: They're reviewing the list; they're calling the patients to come in for their A1Cs [a type of blood test] or come in for their colonoscopies or whatever. It can't just be at the doctor visit that this happens. . . . We have to create a structure around the doc so the care management happens and it gets the doc working at the top of his or her license as opposed to trying to be doing everything him- or herself.
>
> —practice administrator, large multispecialty practice

Similarly, one hospital leader described how ACO care management teams generated cost savings by focusing on socioeconomic barriers to care:

> To be honest, we have not seen that the interventions within the walls of the physician office make all that much difference in a shared savings model, when you're looking at dollars saved. . . . Where we generate the shared savings is once the patient leaves the office. It is the care management models around that patient. It is determining [the patient's] socioeconomic determinants of health care. . . . And those aren't usually due to poor medical decisionmaking in the office. . . . It's because [the patient] didn't get [a] prescription filled. . . . [The patient] didn't have transportation to get back to the doctor's office, so it was easier to call 911 or come to the [emergency room]. . . .
>
> —CEO, hospital participating in an ACO with local physician practices

For primary care practices of multiple sizes and ownership models, the care management activities encouraged by medical home programs required investment in new staff members. One such respondent described it this way:

> [The medical home] created a lot more work. . . . We had to retrofile the patients. . . . Our highest-risk patients, after we stratify them; they come in; we have to do a care plan. My staff spends an extra 15 or 20 minutes going over goals for them to do. . . . We spend more time with our structured way of going over all screening tests. We send letters to people who aren't up to date. We track referrals, which we weren't doing before. Most of it is staff. . . . I had to hire probably equal to about one and a half staff people to be able to do all of that.
>
> —physician, solo primary care practice participating in medical home and episode-based payment programs

Changes in Access
Alternative payment models that reward care management were described as encouraging physician practices to enhance their accessibility outside of regular business hours. In one market,

an observer reported that this change would be a significant departure from the current community standard among many physicians:

> In this market, when physicians go home [from] their office, it's really hard to get a hold of them on the phone. . . . If you call their office after hours with a problem, you're going to get a recording that says, "This is our office hours, and, if you have a medical emergency, go to the emergency room. Otherwise, call us tomorrow." That's going to need to change to manage care differently . . . because people aren't just sick 8 to 5.
>
> —leader, medical society

Alternative payment models have prompted practices to offer alternative ways to access physicians and other clinicians, such as patient portals and mobile care units, to extend care delivery into patients' communities. As one physician practice participating in shared savings and capitation explained,

> Certain communities need services provided in the community because certain patients, we've learned from our Medicaid and [other safety-net] experience that oftentimes patients are reluctant to go to the hospital for various reasons . . . yet the patients and their families still have issues that need to be addressed. So we'll deploy a mobile unit to a community center and provide care there . . . to make sure we are managing that patient there.
>
> —physician leader, medium-sized, single-specialty practice

Changing Relationships Between Physicians

Practice respondents and all types of market observers across study markets noted alternative payment models to have affected relationships between primary care physicians and other specialists in multiple ways. Most frequently, this was reported by primary care practices, likely because respondents perceived that most performance measures and patient-attribution methods were based on primary care activities.

In particular, global capitation and virtual global capitation (via shared savings) have realigned incentives to encourage greater cooperation between primary care physicians and other specialists:

> Most of these [shared savings program] measurements are based on either cost metrics or safety metrics that are aimed at preventing [patients from] needing a surgeon. But not too many of them that I know of are based on how good of a job the surgeon does. . . . It's cheaper for your organization if you manage blood pressure better, diabetes better . . . because there's going to be [fewer] heart attacks and strokes and all that. . . . We've set up a team . . . to interface better with [our internists] to see if specialists can help . . . try and avoid getting the asthmatic to need pulmonary [specialists.] There's a feeling in our organization that the specialists were not invested enough earlier on, and we're trying to sort of bridge that gap. . . .
>
> —subspecialist physician, large multispecialty practice participating in PFP, shared savings, and medical home programs

Some subspecialists reported better professional satisfaction as a consequence of greater collaboration with primary care physicians. For example, a psychiatrist who previously had been "carved out" of nearly all payment models previously applied to his medical group reported feeling rejuvenated by a global shared savings payment model that included his specialty, enabling him to make new contributions to patient care as part of an interdisciplinary team that included primary care physicians and health coaches:

> [The current shared savings contract] is the first thing I'm not carved out of. . . . Somebody finally decided, "You know, behavioral health has a lot of influence on medical outcomes." [So we have] implemented collaborative care in a bunch of medical practices to find patients who have diabetes, hypertension, cardiac problems, and some mental health comorbidities and see if it was possible to improve adherence and outcomes if we fine-tune their [mental health] care. [I go] to several different internal medicine practices and . . . the health coach presents a patient, the [primary care physician] talks about what's going on, and I would say . . . "We could optimize that antidepressant regimen in the following way," . . . Or, I would say, "There's substantial evidence now that they have a paranoid psychosis, and this is not something a [primary care physician] should try to manage. We need to get somebody else in there." . . . I think this is a good idea. I think it's good for patients. I enjoy being with these health coaches, and seeing their eagerness to acquire knowledge and be effective is cool.
>
> —psychiatrist, large network with PFP, shared savings, and capitation

Despite many instances of improved relationships between primary care physicians and other specialists, tensions could arise from a fundamental shift for subspecialty care: In FFS payment, subspecialty care contributed to practice revenue; but in global capitation and shared savings programs, subspecialty care was instead a cost to the practice (similar to hospital care). This change in status could be uncomfortable for some subspecialists. As this respondent explained,

> This new paradigm, to some extent, creates a little bit of a divide because you've got your primary care physicians who are being tasked with kind of controlling cost in some way, and they do referrals to specialists for different procedures, etc., and then you've got the specialists who are feeling that all of the attention and stick-banging is being done to them.
>
> —leader, medical society

Both primary care physicians and subspecialist physicians in multiple markets reported that alternative payment models encouraging cost containment had prompted some physicians to limit care provided outside their organizations (i.e., "stopping leakage"), thus changing referral relationships. One respondent reported,

> What it changed is that now we're much tougher in sending people out of the system. . . . Because any place you go it's going to be more expensive than to do the stuff here. . . . I tell people that, "If you want to have us manage your care, you can't have your stuff scattered all over town."
>
> —primary care physician, solo practice in an ACO

Comparison Between Current Findings and Previously Published Research

Findings from the current study correlate with existing literature indicating that administrative burdens are increased when practices participate in PFP (Halladay et al., 2009) and that medical home and ACO models require the addition of new staff, such as care coordinators and care managers (Burns and Pauly, 2012; Peikes et al., 2014), and encourage teamwork (Bitton, Schwartz, et al., 2012). We did not identify empirical research exploring the influence of the alternative payment models included in the current study on relationships between physicians.

CHAPTER SEVEN

Increased Importance of Data and Data Analysis

Overview of Findings

In response to alternative payment models, physician practices reported making significant investments in their data management capabilities. Data required for successful participation in alternative payment models consisted of internal data from the practice, usually from an EHR documenting patient care activities, and external data, generally consisting of claims data and claim-based measures reported back to the practice by health plans.

In practices with more–highly developed data management capabilities, several leaders and physicians reported lacking the timely, accurate data they needed to respond to alternative payment models effectively. When present, these data deficiencies were a source of considerable frustration. By far the greatest concerns about data were the potential mismatch between data internal to a practice, from the EHR, reflecting "what actually happened" to the patient, and external data, from payers' claims data, reflecting what was documented for billing purposes. Overall, practice leaders trusted their internal EHR data more than they trusted external data, which they felt were at least one step removed from the "source of truth." Accordingly, internal data often guided practices' QI efforts, even though external data frequently served as the basis for alternative payment models (e.g., PFP bonuses based on claims data).

Although one important goal of alternative payment models is to achieve cost savings over a traditional FFS system, ironically, respondents noted that accurate cost data could be difficult to obtain, especially accurate price data for health care services and commodities (e.g., specialty drugs). When data on prices were unavailable, this limited practices' abilities to contain the costs of care—as encouraged in alternative payment models, such as capitation, shared savings, and episode-based and bundled payments. This nonavailability of price data was attributed, in some cases, to some health plans' unwillingness to share such data with physicians, perhaps because of confidentiality and agreements with pharmaceutical and device companies regarding rebates or discounts.

Respondents expressed varying degrees of frustration with their ability to enter data into their own internal data systems. There was no clear consistency in the practices that exhibited greater or lesser comfort with this task—in our sample, there were small, independent, solo practitioners who felt they were able to enter their data and manage them well, and there were large, hospital-owned practices that had experienced great frustrations with entering and managing their own internal data. Practices reported making significant investments in their data management capabilities, ranging from adopting or upgrading EHRs to committing physician and staff time and effort to data entry, management, and analysis.

Detailed Findings

Concerns About Existing Data Sources

Physician practices and hospital leaders frequently reported that data they received from external sources were not timely, limiting their usefulness for the purpose of improving performance in alternative payment models. This was reported by a wide variety of practices and market observers, in nearly all study markets, but most frequently by medium-sized and large practices that possessed greater capabilities to analyze such data than smaller practices had. Delays in data provided to physician practices can limit the usefulness of these data for guiding practice improvements, as described here:

> We're not getting timely and complete data. . . . By the time the information's provided to [physician practices], it's sometimes eight to 14 months old. And so it's really kind of hard to use that as opportunities for discussions about changing practice patterns.
>
> —leader, hospital system with affiliated physician practices

In another practice that participated in shared savings programs with multiple payers, performance data from one payer were continually being corrected and arriving late, making it difficult for the practice to monitor its own performance and make timely course corrections:

> What is frustrating is that [the health plan] changes its mind all the time; the data they give you [are] bad; they give you something and then they say, "No, it's wrong. We're going to give you something else." You don't ever feel comfortable that what they say today is going to be true tomorrow. . . . And the fact that the data [come] in so late that it isn't always clear whether you're making money or not and what the issues are is very distressing. . . .
>
> —leader, large multispecialty practice

Even when practices received bonus payments, several practice leaders reported receiving few usable data on how performance could be improved. Respondents most often cited such payment models as PFP as models in which payers might simply send a bonus check (or not) to the practice at the end of the reporting period, with few useful data on how practices might improve. Because these payment models were often associated with relatively modest incentives, it was particularly frustrating for physician practices to expend time and energy to collect the data while not feeling that there was an upside benefit. This respondent described feedback received from a PFP program:

> Unfortunately, the way that we get our reporting on that, it's very unclear. Like, I want to see transparency. I want to know what we're not doing that we're not getting the dollars for. Or what we're doing right that we are getting the dollars for. And it's really hard to find that information out. I usually, we get a [PFP bonus] check, then I call and say, "Okay, what measures did we meet? Where is it coming from? What's our new measures?" . . . And sometimes you don't get the answer.
>
> —practice manager, small single-specialty practice

In response to such concerns and to improve the likelihood that their alternative payment models would succeed, some health plan leaders we interviewed described developing programs to provide practices with timely, regular data and, moreover, with customized guidance in how to use these data to improve their performance. This respondent described providing such data and support to participants in the plan's bundled payment and medical home models:

> We gather claims data and report [them] out to the providers on a quarterly basis so that they can see how they're performing. . . . We will have our medical directors sit down and walk through the reports with them, explain it to them, answer questions, and help point out ways where, "Here's where you're less efficient compared to these other groups, and [here are] changes you can make to get more in line. [Here are] things that we see other groups doing differently than you're doing."
>
> —leader, health plan

We note that, in this particular market and concerning this particular health plan, physician practices did not report the kinds of data concerns heard elsewhere.

Although Internal Data Might Theoretically Be More Readily Available, These Data Are Largely Drawn from Electronic Health Records, Raising Issues with Ease of Data Extraction and Integration

Respondents described numerous difficulties with the complexities of extracting and managing data from their own EHRs and related recordkeeping systems. Even when all data were in electronic format, there were problems with data integration, formatting, and compatibility. Practices with greater resources, such as those that were part of larger health systems, seemed better able to address these challenges. However, some larger organizations faced the problem of consolidating data from multiple EHRs:

> We have a total of about 26 different EMR [electronic medical record] systems, so probably every one you can think of out there is out there, and then some you haven't heard of are out there. . . . We're building a centralized data warehouse . . . where we have pay-for-performance contracts; we already get data feeds from the payers. . . . We're also beginning to integrate EMR data into that as well. . . . We do want to connect all of our primary care physicians, all of those specialists [who] take care of chronic disease. . . . It's hard enough to get data out of them, even though they may be meaningful use. It is a very difficult thing to do. . . .
>
> —director, IPA

In other instances, the disruption of having recently changed to a new EHR required staff to relearn fundamental data-extraction techniques:

> The changes in the world kind of make you—you're kind of like a tornado coming along and everything's scattered and you have to put it all back together and start over again. . . . We have to really get our EMR back in shape and be able to pull data out of it so that we can know what we're doing right and what we're doing wrong.
>
> —physician leader, medium-sized primary care practice

Data Used by Payers to Calculate Potential Payments as Part of Alternative Payment Models Do Not Always Agree with the Data That Practices Are Using Internally to Track Performance

Payers most often use data external to the practice (claims or billing data) to calculate a practice's performance on measures underlying an alternative payment model. These data, even when derived from practice EHRs that also serve as billing software, are frequently not equivalent to the data that practices are using internally to track performance. These differences can stem from documentation and billing challenges rather than patient care. For example, in the instance of payment models that reward processes of care, EHRs could permit a single process to be documented in a variety of different ways, but not all documentation methods will generate the CPT code required for the practice to accurately report the services that a physician provided. Such frustrations were described by respondents in practices of all specialties and in all markets, and most prominently by small and primary care practices participating in PFP programs and some episode-based payment programs.

This respondent described the process of identifying inaccuracies in payer-provided reports in a PFP model:

> It's a lot of resolving mismatches. So [the health plan] sends us, "Here are your scores," and we say, "Well, based on our EHR data, [the scores are different]." So we're trying to figure out why things don't match. . . . We order the mammogram; we get it documented in our EHR; for whatever reason, it doesn't end up in the health plan files. . . . If you document the mammogram, [on] the clinical side, they did the right thing, whether the health plan records it or not. . . . Because that's more accurate, that's actually what happened to the patient, versus what, for whatever reason, get picked up in the coding, which is presumably less accurate.
>
> —physician, large multispecialty practice

Another respondent described inaccuracies in payers' data about which physicians were in the practice, leading to mistakes in utilization data on imaging studies:

> A huge insurance company [came] over here with [its] data wanting to discuss, "Well, doctor, this is what you're doing." Well, guess what? [Its] data had doctors [who] aren't even in my group and doctors [who] had left the group years ago. So [those are] the data that they are presenting to me, so you question the accuracy. . . . Or they said, "Listen, you're referring too many x-rays to such and such a place," and I've never even heard of such and such a place. . . . This is one of the bigger, more-sophisticated insurance companies, [yet] I'm not sure if their data [are accurate].
>
> —physician leader, small single-specialty practice

Complete and Accurate Data on Costs of Components of Care Can Be Difficult to Obtain, Limiting Physicians' Abilities to Contain Health Care Costs

Although overall data accuracy was a frequently cited concern from physician practices with regard to existing data sources, data about costs seemed particularly difficult to obtain. These concerns were voiced by respondents in nearly all markets, but notably, they were not expressed by small practices or primary care practices in this study—perhaps because such practices were less likely to participate in payment models that put them at risk for global costs of care (thereby increasing the importance of cost data). Incomplete data on drug costs were noted as an area of particular concern:

> [Drug A] is a drug that costs about $25,000 a year for the treatment of [disease]. It has about a 50-percent response rate. If a patient is failing that, you can double the dose, and you can get probably [a] 60-percent response rate. You compare that to [drug B], and you start out with a 69-percent response rate, right, at essentially $25,000. So in an era where you . . . care what the cost is . . . you start to think, "Well, they're pretty much equivalent, so maybe I should switch the [drug A] double-dose people over to the single dose of [drug B], because I'm bringing down the cost by half." But then what gets interjected, which makes this complicated, is there's all these backroom deals that insurers have with the drug companies. So I actually don't really know if making that substitution actually saves any money at the end of the day. . . . I don't have the right information. . . . I've tried to get it from multiple different vantage points, and I can't get it.
>
> —physician leader, large multispecialty practice

Respondents also noted that, when cost data are made available, such data can be effective tools for changing physician behavior:

> Just two days ago, I got a report of cholecystectomy costs broken down by physician, by group, by what everything costs, and we've said this for a long time: "If you will tell a physician what something really costs and show them what impact they can make, then they will make the decision as to whether or not that's important enough for them to continue to use or not to use it." . . . One of the things is that, for cholecystectomy, I have hung on a long time to a dissection tool that is my preference; it's called a harmonic scalpel, but . . . they told me . . . "This is how much more it costs, and this is where you are compared to the other physicians in the cost per case." . . . I got rid of the harmonic scalpel.
>
> —physician leader, small single-subspecialty practice participating in an episode-based payment program

Investments in Data Infrastructure

In order to generate, understand, and take action in many alternative payment models, a wide variety of respondents within and outside physician practices in all markets explained that practices required significant data management infrastructures. Some practices tended to be flexible in describing how such infrastructure could be achieved, whether through a practice's own initiative, through support from other practices or IPAs, or from a hospital or payer:

> Data [are] important. You don't have to have your own data warehouse. You can use the data that the payer gives you and work with [them]. But you have to have information to understand where your high-risk patients are, what your performance metrics are. . . . Or you have to pay someone to get [those] data to you.
>
> —physician leader, large multispecialty practice

Other practices, especially smaller and primary care practices, struggled to keep up with new data management needs and hesitated to make specific investments because of uncertainty about future participation in alternative payment models:

> The data management is a huge, huge piece of [whether to participate in alternative payment models.] It's a full-time job as a practice manager to just manage that data reporting. . . . I'd either have had to hire a consultant to help write it, or it comes out of your hide. You're doing it on Saturdays and Sundays.
>
> —practice administrator, medium-sized primary care practice participating in medical home and episode-based programs

Although off-the-shelf data systems are tempting for their ease of use, multiple practices employing them reported ongoing problems. Conversely, practices that had built customized data solutions reported expending large amounts of financial and human capital in the development process but also had systems that were then responsive to their specific needs and workflows. For example, this practice administrator, whose practice had been participating in an episode-based, bundled payment model for a little more than a year, emphasized the foundational work required to participate in the payment model:

> Data collection was a big deal for us. . . . We weren't even tracking how many CHF [congestive heart failure] admissions we had. We knew how many readmissions we had, and we thought we had our hands around numerators and denominators, but we weren't exactly sure. The data had never really been validated really hard, and so we had to look to our folks both in health information management, our enterprise data warehouse, analysts within the organization to . . . determine where our sources for data were. . . . It really was a big onion that we had to peel away a layer at a time.
>
> —practice administrator, small single-specialty practice participating in an episode-based, bundled payment program

Data Entry

Practices participating in alternative payment models, particularly those with high documentation requirements, such as medical homes programs and bundled or episode-based payments, placed increased importance on accurate and systematic data entry. This was noted broadly by both practice and hospital respondents, and more commonly in small practices and primary care practices. We note that respondents from surgical subspecialty practices did not report on the importance of data entry, potentially because fewer performance measures applied to such practices.

Data entry was described as a task that was often distributed among multiple individuals within a practice, including front-office staff, MAs, nurses, mid-levels, and physicians. In smaller practices, data entry often fell to physicians alone, while larger practices had support, such as scribes, or MAs, who took on the bulk of necessary documentation. One respondent, whose practice was participating in medical home and episode-based payment programs, explained,

> Probably the biggest significant difference is there's been a real push on the physicians to make sure that they're following best practice and also that they are documenting in a way that we can do reporting so that we can take a look at managing the population, so that we can pull out who's one of our diabetics . . . so the biggest change, I think, has really been pushing the providers to make sure that they're documenting in a way that we can then find information so that we can do care management and so that we can do better quality control . . . so that we can follow up with them and keep on top of them.
>
> —practice administrator, medium-sized primary care practice

Perhaps recognizing that physicians who are paid based on productivity within the practice will lose revenue if they spend too much time on documentation tasks, some practices were able to pay physicians to collect data that were vital to risk adjustment in alternative payment models. In this example, an IPA participating in an ACO program provided its primary care physicians with additional fee-for-documentation revenue as a way to enable physicians to invest more time in documenting patients' diagnoses:

> We actually prepaid them to fill out a health risk-assessment form so we could find out more about these patients because we really didn't know anything about these patients other than what Medicare had given us. And so, part of their bonus was a prepaid bonus and that, "Here, we're going to pay you a fee-for-service on top of your visit for giving us information on the patients." . . . That alone was a huge value to the physician and frankly to the patient, having all that information aggregated in one place.
>
> —physician leader, IPA

Physicians Are Not Averse to Entering Data Differently If They Perceive That They Can Have an Effect on Clinical Care for Patients, but They Express Frustration When Asked to Spend Time on Data Entry Simply to Meet a Perceived Documentation Need

Despite widespread concern among our respondents about the amount of time required for data entry in alternative payment models, physicians appreciate that some data-entry requirements have changed and improved patient care. Physicians from a variety of practices seemed largely willing and, in some cases, even excited to be able to better monitor patients and provide better care through activities enabled by data entry. However, when physicians perceived that they were being asked to spend significant amounts of time purely for documentation purposes, they were more likely to express annoyance:

> I think some [data entry is] useful, [but] some of it is excess work to do to get population data to manage costs for insurance companies. . . . It's useful if it can [help you] recall information that you need when you need it for patients, such as they need a pap smear or they need a lipid panel or they need a this or a that. Or it can be very useful for maybe coming up with conflicts, such as medication interactions and things like that. I think a lot of the data entry that we do on a daily basis is not useful. . . . Clicking "mark as reviewed" for problem lists and medication lists is not useful. . . . It's just clicking a box that you can get

meaningful-use paid to say you do it. . . . It's just a way that they can document that you do something.

—physician leader, medium-sized primary care practice participating in episode-based and medical home programs

Activities Enabled by Data and Data Analysis

In spite of the challenges to data entry, management, and analysis, nearly all categories of respondents across all study markets were able to identify activities that were possible only as a result of the data that had been collected, reviewed, or analyzed in order to meet the requirements of various alternative payment models.

Care Management Activities Made Possible Using Data That Practices Collect as Part of Their Participation in Alternative Payment Models

Current data capabilities have allowed practices to do something as seemingly simple as create a registry of their patients. Newly available data have improved care management abilities, allowing for more-granular detail on the patient population, as described by this respondent implementing a shared savings model:

> I think our ability to use data analytics is far superior than it was in the '90s. So, our ability to segment patients into categories that allow us to better focus on what the needs are. . . . 20 percent of the people spend 80 percent of the dollars. The difficulty in the 1990s is you couldn't find those 20 percent of the people until they had already spent the money. Now, we find them through the use of data and data analytics, biometric screening, prospective assessments. . . . We didn't have those tools back in the '90s. So much of what managed care was done retrospectively and was done in a scarcity or a rationing model. I like to talk about our current model of care as being more of an abundance model. We want to provide abundantly to the needs of the population. . . . That certainly doesn't mean inappropriate. That just means for what they need, abundance.

—leader, hospital

Another form of care management might include being able to provide care in alternative settings or using alternative modalities. This respondent described how data drove the development of an alternative mode of care delivery:

> We monitor and measure pretty much anything and everything, and certain trends identify a need. In this specific instance, it wasn't hard. We noticed that, for this patient population, the [Medicare Supplement Insurance] or Medicaid patient population, that the no-show rate was very high, and yet we knew the patient had problems, conditions—endocarditis, discharged with [a myocardial infarction], malignant hypertension. . . . We know and understand when a trend is not right. So the first clue was the no-show rate.

—physician leader, medium-sized single-specialty practice

Data Collected, Analyzed, and Reported to Practices as a Result of Participation in Alternative Payment Models Provide Valuable (and Often Appreciated) Feedback to Physicians

Despite some concerns regarding the timeliness, complexity, and accuracy of data, a wide variety of respondents from almost all study markets appreciated feedback when it was able to direct meaningful improvements in patient care. Some respondents noted that, before they received such feedback, they had believed they were providing high-quality care, but, when the data indicated otherwise, they appreciated having direction for making improvements:

> In general, if you don't track it, most doctors think they did a marvelous job, and then when you track it, they find out that they're way less than what they really thought they would be. . . . A lot of that kind of stuff can fall by the wayside. We have medical assistants and nurses . . . and doctors all looking for those things or reliability in getting them done . . . like their patients are getting their A1Cs more frequently. . . . I think that the doctors are happy that it happened.

> —physician leader, large multispecialty practice

Although feedback based on individual physician performance, or the performance of a single practice, was appreciated as a tool for assessing quality and making potential improvements to patient care, there was also a distinct appreciation for external data that could allow for benchmarking across organizations and sometimes across geographic regions, as described by this respondent:

> The number of reports has expanded dramatically. The sophistication and clarity of them has expanded. The ability to drill down. . . . One of the important things is they see their performance compared to all the other physician organizations in the state. So, it's not just "How are we doing internally in our community?" . . . It's more, "How are they doing compared to the range of performance amongst their peers?" . . . There are some that perform really well. So, we show in a current real world what can be accomplished.

> —leader, health plan

Data on Performance Are Increasingly Being Gathered, Analyzed, and Interpreted with a View Toward How the Public Will View the Results

Many respondents were aware that many performance data will eventually be publicly reported, and they had an eye toward being able to use such data to attract more patients or otherwise help their organizations stand out in a crowded health care market. This practice leader strategized that overall value would become increasingly important under alternative payment models. High performance could be used to communicate the practice's value to patients and consumers:

> I think overall everyone is much more aware that our value has to be demonstrated. And so the question of why should I come to you instead of going somewhere else or why should I come to you and have a huge copay, why should I come to you and not go to Minute Clinic, those types of—kind of the value proposition, we're getting pushed much harder to

articulate, and I think that providers are much more aware of that than they've ever been, even in this context where we feel like we're a very special provider.

—practice leader, large multispecialty practice

This physician expressed excitement at the now-aligned incentives within the system, to provide better care while emphasizing efficiency:

The old managed care thing, yeah. That was really all about ratcheting down availability of care for people. That really wasn't about making them healthier. Nobody was talking about, "This is good for you." They were only talking about, "You can't have that test because it's too expensive." So, to me, it is quite different even though it sort of feels the same in some ways. . . . It's good business for people to be healthy. We finally figured that out. . . . I really feel like really for the first time, the focus is on the right thing. . . . It's never really been like that. It's really been like have the nicest lobby and, you know, have the prettiest building and buy the latest scanner. All that stuff definitely counts, but I love the fact that all of [these] data [are] publicly reported. You have never seen hospitals and doctors scramble like they're scrambling now until you see them have people go to healthcare. gov and be able to look up their infection rate for total [knee replacements]. I mean that is spectacular. I love that.

—solo primary care practitioner

Comparison Between Current Findings and Previously Published Research

There was little existing literature specifically examining the influence of payment models on the need to develop a greater role for data. The most relevant existing literature was related to administrative needs. PFP has been shown to increase administrative burden and reporting requirements, particularly for smaller practices, and practices serving patients from many different health plans (Halladay et al., 2009). However, the study did not attempt to measure the subset of "administrative burden and reporting requirements" related specifically to data acquisition, management, and analysis.

There is some support in existing literature for our finding that, in some instances, it will be necessary to build system capacity to manage, share, and analyze data. Several studies have found that technical assistance from payers to providers participating in ACO programs can improve provider capabilities, data sharing systems, and joint strategic planning via close provider–payer relationships (Higgins et al., 2011; Claffey et al., 2012; Larson et al., 2012). Finally, we did not identify studies that quantified the investments in data management and analytic capacity made by physician practices in order to participate and succeed in alternative payment models.

CHAPTER EIGHT

Interactions Among Payment Programs and Between Payment Programs and Government Regulations

Overview of Findings

In a pluralistic health care system, typical physician practices have contracts with a variety of different health plans, each of which applies its own payment model. In this context, the effects of each health plan's payment model might depend not only on the model itself but also on how it interacts with the payment models used by the other payers.

One clear finding from our interviews was that the multiplicity of PFP and other incentive programs has created a heavy administrative burden on some physician practices. Merely keeping track of payment program details, which vary from payer to payer, required management effort that could be beyond the capacity of some practices. In response, larger physician practices and hospital systems have stepped into the role of boiling those incentives down into something that is more manageable, and palatable, for their physicians.

Performance incentives offered by multiple payers could reinforce each other, and incentives from one payer led, in some cases, to practice-wide changes affecting all of the practice's patients. But a serious tension could also arise when practices participate in a mix of both FFS and risk-based contracts. In these situations, practices faced fundamentally conflicting incentives—to increase volume under the FFS contract while reducing costs under the risk-based contract. This conflict was especially acute for hospital-owned physician practices, in which reductions in hospital utilization—which are strongly incentivized under risk-based contracts—could undermine the financial well-being of the parent organization. Resolving those conflicts required striking a careful balance and seeking population health initiatives that controlled total costs without sabotaging the FFS revenue stream.

In addition, multiple practices described spillover effects from the EHR installations and upgrades encouraged by meaningful-use incentives. In some cases, EHRs had positive effects, facilitating the achievement of performance targets in PFP and shared savings programs. In other cases, especially when new EHRs replaced legacy systems, some interviewees described significant setbacks in their ability to meet the goals of these alternative payment programs.

Detailed Findings

Administrative Challenges
Multiple Sets of Performance Metrics Create Burdens
The typical physician practice accepts patients from multiple payers, including multiple commercial plans, Medicare FFS, Medicare Advantage, and Medicaid. The multiplicity of payers

has always created complexities for physician practices in their billing and collections and regulatory compliance. But, with PFP incentives and other alternative payment models becoming more common, physician practices across all markets, particularly large and medium practices, that might have greater capacity than small practices to participate in multiple different payment models, reported heavy administrative burdens from the growing cacophony of metrics:

> One of the challenges is [that every health plan] has different gates and different metrics. And so for practices, that's a real challenge in terms of . . . taking risks from maybe three or four different payers and yet we're being measured differently by each one of those payers. And so the need for uniformity around quality measures or metrics is critical.
>
> —leader, medical society

Respondents pointed out that, in some cases, there was a valid rationale for applying different performance metrics to different plans. Control targets for diabetes differ for the elderly versus nonelderly, for example. But, more often, respondents cited a multiplicity of metrics and reporting methods with no clear clinical rationale:

> When you ask what the biggest stress for our primary care practices [is], it's the fact that we're not just moving them to patient-centered medical homes; . . . the stress is trying to figure out how to manage all these quality metrics.
>
> —leader, large IPA

Different Players Are Stepping Up to Filter and Harmonize Performance Metrics

Respondents explained that the profusion of performance metrics creates two problems for physician practices. The first problem is that physicians cannot reasonably be expected to be aware of and adhere to an overwhelming number of metrics. The second problem is that physicians reported flawed use of some metrics, either because these metrics are clinically off-target or because the administrative burden is disproportionate to the financial reward. Addressing those problems requires filtering performance metrics—i.e., deciding which ones are worth paying any attention to and which are not—and harmonizing performance metrics—i.e., boiling a large number of metrics down to a simpler performance standard that can be communicated to and comprehended by practicing clinicians. Within our sample, several types of organizations have stepped up and taken leadership roles in synchronizing performance metrics, including hospital systems, large physician practices, medical societies, and locally dominant health plans.

For physician practices, a first step in filtering and harmonizing performance metrics is simply to catalog those that are currently in place, which requires some management effort. A leader from a medium-sized physician practice described the development of a "crossover document" that identified the commonalities among CMS's meaningful-use program (a federal program to encourage EHR adoption by physician practices) and various medical home programs. One respondent described a similar process:

> We've taken all the quality measures from our payers and put them on this giant spreadsheet [to identify] where are payers looking at similar things.

> —leader, large PHO

Some smaller practices disregarded performance metrics that they perceived as not worth the administrative hassle. Larger practices also chose consciously to disregard metrics that they perceived as invalid, sometimes simultaneously adopting supplemental metrics not required by plans because they aligned with their missions or were relevant to their specific patient populations:

> If we think [that a performance metric] is stupid, we won't do it. . . . We've also incentivized things that the [payer] doesn't look at. For example, [for] our population, we think that domestic violence screening is something really important, and that's not something we do [for] pay for performance; it's something we believe in.

> —leader, large primary care practice

Some large practices and IPAs also reported pressuring health plans during contract negotiations to apply a common set of performance metrics, although with mixed success:

> The biggest thing that we try to work on [in negotiating risk contracts] is mostly to get the quality [measurement] component to be similar, and, to be perfectly honest, we've given up because it just doesn't happen.

> —leader, large IPA

Hospital systems have the administrative resources to undertake the work of filtering and harmonizing metrics, and they are able to set compensation parameters for their employed physicians and the practices they own. As a result, some hospital systems have stepped squarely into the role of filtering and harmonizing performance metrics:

> Our intent . . . was to have a single report card for the entire network. The doctors know exactly what metrics they're being held accountable to, and they don't have to say, "well, gosh, you're a [payer A] patient, so I have to do these metrics." And "you're a [payer B] patient, so I had to do this set of metrics. . . ."

> —leader, hospital

Conflicting Incentives
Fee-for-Service Incentives Fundamentally at Odds with Incentives in Other Payment Models

The FFS payment arrangement embeds a very simple financial incentive—produce more units of service—that conflicts with the incentives under alternative payment arrangements. Respondents in larger practices in markets in which capitation (and virtual capitation through shared savings) was common described the tension their practices faced from treating patients paid under a mix of FFS and alternative payment models, as exemplified by the following respondent:

> [Payment] had been basically fee-for-service and very volume oriented, and we had to make a shift to pay more attention to what the managed care plans were picking for us to improve upon. . . . People use the [expression] "One foot in each of two canoes"—one fee-for-service leg and one [in a] value-based performance contract.
>
> —physician leader, large multispecialty practice

Another respondent pointed out conflict arising from competing time pressures:

> We have a real problem since most of the market is still volume-driven and . . . many of the [medical home program] things that are required slow down the physician and, therefore, cost the physician the ability to see patients.
>
> —leader, small primary care practice

Hospital systems in multiple markets noted a more profound conflict between their risk-sharing and capitation contracts, which reward reductions in total spending, and their FFS revenue, which is heavily driven by hospital utilization. One executive described the situation as "looking in both directions":

> [We are] trying to build systems in which we in fact create incentives for more-thoughtful and appropriate utilization; the latter being very inspiring around patient care because, when you see reductions in readmission rates and more-appropriate utilization, it's terrific, but, when you see basically empty beds and reductions in utilization that challenge [hospital] revenue, it puts more-rapid cost pressure on unit costs and makes it harder to kind of think through how to keep the incentives aligned.
>
> —leader, hospital

Practices Seek Initiatives That Meet Multiple Goals

Setting management priorities under disparate and sometimes-conflicting incentives has been likened to "threading a really thin needle." All types of practice respondents and market observers in all markets described the importance (and difficulty) of aligning the goals of various payment models. One respondent described seeking and prioritizing opportunities to meet multiple goals, rather than wading into areas likely to involve trade-offs between competing goals:

> The place where we're able to get the most traction is when we can find a quality or patient and family experience issue that can be addressed that has, like, the positive externality of also supporting our [total cost] initiatives.
>
> —physician leader, large multispecialty practice

One approach to reconciling conflicting payment incentives is to focus on reducing the utilization and costs of services provided outside the organization that bears the risk. For physician-owned groups, the obvious place to look is utilization of hospital services or drugs. For hospital-owned practices, however, a narrower range of services is in play:

> What do you want to get rid of in your population management? You want [to get rid of] high-cost, low-margin . . . things that don't affect your practice, [such as] the drugs that you use. . . . That's the first thing that you [target for reduction]. Labs and ancillaries, potentially if they're not within network also . . . that is someone else's bottom line as opposed to your own. And what you're going to hold onto is anything that is high margin but low cost, . . . because that's what keeps [your own] operation going.

—leader, large multispecialty practice

Positive Reinforcements and Spillovers
One Payer's Incentives Can Spill Over to Affect Other Payers' Patients

For practical and ethical reasons, physician practices reported generally applying the same treatment protocols to all patients. This was reported in several markets by practices of all sizes, specialties, and ownership models. As a result, some practices reported that an alternative payment model used by one payer was having spillover effects on treatment of enrollees in FFS plans. For example, a physician leader in a Medicare ACO described care management services as one of the key responses to participating in an ACO—but those services were made available to all high-risk patients in the practice, not just those in the Medicare ACO panel. Another respondent in a medical home described a similarly broad initiative:

> We're [creating a care plan] for every patient [who] walks in the door, whether they're Medicaid or Medicare or [commercial payer,] because that's part of what we do . . . , because we think that's what a [medical home] does.

—leader, primary care practice

This respondent described a practice that had a PFP contract with one payer, but the workflows developed to respond to that incentive affected all patients in the practice:

> The assumption is, when a patient is in an exam room and the physician is in there, they're not really concentrating on who the payer is; [the doctor is] examining the patient, [the patient's] problem, diagnosing, and setting a treatment plan. . . . So if [the doctor is] made aware of an opportunity and there is sound medical reason behind that opportunity, and [the doctor] already [knows] that . . . using generics when available makes perfectly good sense—You know what? It's not so much even the compensation; it's just, "this makes sense. . . ."

—leader, medical society

Electronic Health Records Have Enabled Better Performance Under Pay for Performance and Risk-Based Contracting

Respondents from all study markets and practice types described certain positive effects of EHR adoption, which was spurred by meaningful-use requirements and other local programs.

For some practices, EHR adoption helped practices improve performance under alternative payment models. For example, one respondent reported this:

> If all the physicians get onboard to standards of care and benchmarks, that's much easier to do with an EHR, because you can build your templates to say, "at a certain age, you do blood pressure; you do an EKG; this is for well visits, for example. . . ." So when you're under a risk contract, if you build the EHR templates to order or jog your memory to order, you know exactly what to do for a certain age . . . or a certain chronic disease.
>
> —leader, MGMA chapter

Another respondent noted this:

> We have really good . . . data because we use an EHR that generates reports. . . . I think on the quality data, we really moved the needle in the last three to four years. Our quality scores have gone from below average to really top for safety-net organizations.
>
> —leader, large multispecialty practice

In addition, meaningful-use incentives and EHR adoption can also help practices become accredited as medical homes and help them meet other medical home goals. For example, one respondent participating in a medical home program observed this:

> Since we do have an EMR, . . . we build [documentation] into their templates so that it's right there. . . . So they can click on "Care Plan," they can click on "Asthma," and it can insert the standards of what follow-up for a controlled asthmatic would be, and they will meet the documentation requirements for the care plan. So where possible, we have tried to take advantage of the technology that we already have in place to use it to achieve the new documentation goals so that we're not continually adding 30 seconds here and a minute here and two minutes here to their visit time.
>
> —leader, small primary care practice

Negative Spillover Effects
Disruptions Caused by Changing Electronic Health Records

Respondents in all study markets, including representatives of all physician practice sizes and specialties, also described the negative impacts resulting from EHRs—often immediately following discussion of the positive aspects of EHRs.

As noted earlier, some respondents described instances in which EHR systems were upgraded to meet meaningful-use requirements, causing significant disruption to practice workflows. Some practices had made considerable investments in developing workflows within their original EHRs in response to various payment models. When EHRs needed to be upgraded or changed, these practices' prior investments in building such customizations were lost. This respondent described how an EHR upgrade had disrupted data workflows originally created for meaningful use and a medical home program. Moreover, because the upgrade was part of a larger, system-wide change, it was difficult for the practice to receive priority for rebuilding these workflows within the new EHR:

[The new EHR] undid a lot of stuff that we had done with the previous EHR in terms of workflows. And we still haven't rebuilt all of them. One of those is using prompts for preventive care. . . . We were probably light years ahead of where we are now. . . . What they loaded out of the box for preventive care, it was a catastrophe. . . . the preventive-care module in [old EHR] was configurable. . . . If we decided it was time to start screening for hepatitis C based on the [U.S. Preventive Services Task Force] recommendations, we could add that . . . There was a prompt that we could program in there. . . . [Our new EHR] doesn't have that. . . . What we have now is still not anywhere close to what we need, but that was almost a year ago now, and I'm still asking for support to do that.

—physician leader, medium-sized hospital-owned primary care practice

In other instances, changes initially meant to be beneficial to patients and providers ended up causing more confusion and chaos in the practice. The following respondent described how a practice had recently joined an ACO in which the process of care management was handled by a variety of different individuals, including practice physicians, health plan personnel, and outreach staff from the ACO itself. When roles were not clearly defined, this overlap in responsibilities could cause confusion:

When we entered the ACO . . . we had patients, they could opt out or opt in. . . . It was very unorganized, and I had to hand them these huge packets of information on the ACO. . . . Then you have other insurance companies. . . . They have their mid-level nurse practitioner people that are doing outreach on these patients too. . . . And then what the doctors really, really don't like is that they'll say, "Well, we recommend that you need a diabetic da-da-da." So they call us and they say, "Well, someone called me and I needed a diabetic foot—" . . . They've been worked into a fever pitch, they'll call the doctor and say, "I need this. I want a prescription or the supply. Give it to me." And Dr. [physician name] is like, "Who called you? No, you don't. I need to see you for that. I'm not just going to write you something because—" . . . It can go the opposite way, and then the doctor doesn't even know whether it's the ACO person or whether it's an insurance person doing their outreach, who has even contacted them.

—practice administrator, small primary care practice

Regulations That Inhibit Practices' Ability to Alter Processes of Care

With the exception of physicians practicing in retainer models, respondents in practices of all sizes, specialty, and ownership models described teaming with allied health professionals to help streamline processes of care. However, a small number of respondents reported that state scope-of-practice regulations limited their ability to further optimize the allocation of tasks in response to alternative payment models:

We still face a massive regulatory challenge. . . . I think my medical assistant could talk to the patient and tee up a medical record for me, [but] it's considered out of their scope [of practice]. So [payers are] asking all of these things to happen, but then, again, forcing the physician to personally do them based on scope of practice. And that's going to freeze the progress. . . . They say, "Build the team. Have your MAs help you," and then state law says, "Actually, I'm sorry, they can't."

—physician, large multispecialty practice

Comparison Between Current Findings and Previously Published Research

There is limited prior literature exploring interactions between payment models and between payment models and regulations. However, multiple prior studies have demonstrated spillover effects among payment models, concordant with our finding that, even in practices with several different types of payment models, physicians tend to treat their patients in a consistent way rather than varying their treatment approaches according to payment models employed by each patient's health plan. For example, physicians practicing in geographic areas with high penetration of commercial health plan capitation had lower intensity of care among FFS Medicare beneficiaries (Landon, Reschovsky, O'Malley, et al., 2011), and similar findings were reported for FFS Medicare beneficiaries receiving care from physician groups participating in the Blue Cross and Blue Shield of Massachusetts alternative quality contract (a commercial ACO contract) (McWilliams, Landon, and Chernew, 2013). These findings suggest that physicians in highly capitated practices develop an overall approach to care that also applies to their FFS patients.

CHAPTER NINE

Physician Incentives and Compensation

Overview of Findings

In general, we found that the financial incentives applied to physician practices via alternative payment models were not simply "passed through" to individual physicians. Even practices of relatively modest size reported shielding their physicians from direct exposure to the financial incentives created by payers—except in the case of traditional FFS payment. In fact, the greatest financial incentive facing nearly all physicians in the study, even those in practices with substantial exposure to payment models intended to contain the costs of care (capitation, shared savings, and episode-based payment), was to increase productivity as measured by revenues or RVUs. Notably, only one of the practices in our sample (a solo practice that participated in shared savings) reported having an individual physician compensation formula that included financial rewards for containing the costs of care. Likewise, PFP programs created by payers tended to be simplified by practices before being applied to individual physicians.

This is not to say that physician practices ignored the quality performance or cost-containment incentives they received from payers or sought to insulate individual physicians completely from making changes in response to practice-level financial incentives. Rather, practice leaders described transforming certain practice-level financial incentives (especially those concerning cost containment) into internal nonfinancial incentives for individual physicians, choosing instead to appeal to physicians' intrinsic motivations: professionalism, competitiveness, and desire to improve patient care. Neither upside nor downside cost-based financial incentives were passed to physicians based on their performance as individuals. Common nonfinancial incentives included performance feedback with injunctive norms (in which practice leaders argued for physicians to change their behavior by appealing to sources of authority, such as consensus guidelines) and social norms (in which physicians were shown their performance relative to that of their peers). Some practices also were willing to selectively retain or terminate their physicians based on quality or efficiency performance.

In several practices, leaders acknowledged the presence of inconsistencies between financial and nonfinancial incentives. Barriers to achieving better alignment included a lack of readily available alternatives to RVUs for measuring physician productivity, a desire to avoid dramatic reallocation of income between physicians within the practice, and a need to balance the economic efficiency of physician compensation formulas with practical considerations, such as the operational costs of administering more-complex physician compensation formulas and the trade-off between the complexity and understandability of compensation incentives to physicians.

Generally speaking, alternative payment models had negligible effects on the aggregate income of individual physicians within our sample.

In certain cases, physicians reported wanting to have their incomes more closely linked to quality and efficiency of care. In these cases, physicians expressed an underlying desire to have better alignment between what they thought they should do for patients and what they were paid to do.

Detailed Findings

Financial Incentives for Physicians
Practices Insulate Individual Physician Compensation from Financial Incentives to Contain Costs, Preserving Fee-for-Service Incentives at the Margin

In nearly all practices having significant exposure to alternative payment models (including capitation, shared savings, PFP, and episode-based payment), financial incentives for individual physicians did not mirror closely the financial incentives to the practice. With only one exception (a solo practice that participated in shared savings), none of the 34 practices in our study employed a physician compensation strategy that financially rewarded individual physicians for containing the costs of care—despite approximately half of these practices deriving significant shares of revenues from capitation and shared savings.

As one respondent explained, the practice had decided explicitly to shield individual physicians from financial incentives to contain the costs of care:

> The analogy that I use for this is that, if we've got capitated incentives coming to us as an organization and then we pay doctors a salary that is based on clinical productivity, it's like we have a coat of armor over the physicians that insulates them against these external forces.
>
> —leader, large multispecialty practice with 20 percent of revenue from capitation, shared savings, and PFP programs

Even in practices with substantial risk-based payment, the marginal financial incentive for individual physicians was driven primarily by productivity incentives, with "productivity" measured by RVUs. Nearly all practices in the study—all sizes, specialty, and ownership models and across all study markets—reported that their physicians had this type of individual incentive. Further, for primary care physicians, payments linked to panel sizes also were applied in some cases, but the use of RVUs persisted because of a perceived lack of viable alternatives for measuring individual physician productivity:

> Internal medicine physicians are paid on RVUs and panel sizes. . . . I think we'll have to [use RVUs because] we have to measure productivity somehow. And that's just sort of been the convenient one.
>
> —physician, large multispecialty practice with 75 percent of revenue from capitation and shared savings contracts

For subspecialists, many of whom lacked clear ways to identify their patient panels, RVUs remained the "coin of the realm" and were viewed as a way to monitor these physicians' use of their time, even though practice leaders expressed a desire to avoid unnecessary subspecialist services:

> Frankly, specialists will probably always be incentivized from productivity measures, as well as quality and patient experience. But, you know, their "coin of the realm" is really the units of service. If you think globally, you don't want [specialists] to deliver unnecessary units of service, but that's the way we'll assess whether or not they're effectively using their time. Primary care providers, we've changed it so . . . the real variable component of their incentive is based more on population health outcomes compared to the specialists.
>
> —physician, large multispecialty practice with 30 to 40 percent of revenue from capitation and shared savings contracts

Practices Choose to Apply Financial Incentives for Cost Containment at Higher Organizational Levels

Some practices made payment of bonuses to any individual physician contingent on the overall financial performance of the organization. Although such bonuses were noted broadly by a variety of respondents in all markets, they were most frequently reported by respondents from large, hospital-owned, multispecialty practices. For practices with significant revenues from capitation, this meant that all physicians had a personal financial interest in the efficiency of the practice:

> The entire incentive plan is triggered by a financial trigger [for the practice]. So if we don't hit a certain financial trigger, we don't pay out any incentive to anybody.
>
> —physician, large multispecialty practice with 40 percent capitation, as well as participation in multiple shared savings programs

Other practices retained any earnings under cost-containment incentives, without distribution to individual physicians or triggering any type of payout:

> Every single [payer] gives you bonuses if you meet [its] standards. Like, for example, if you keep [its] patients out of the hospital or if you use the referral system less, [there are] set criteria, and the [practice] as a whole gets the incentive. . . . None of the individual providers here gets any of that.
>
> —physician, large primary care practice

Aside from financial effects, some physicians described other important consequences of practice-level financial performance, such as maintaining adequate staffing levels:

> There's no personal financial incentive at all. There's a global financial effect. I mean, you know, if the group is doing poorly financially, you can't pay—you know, salaries can go

down; you can't hire as many ancillary staff; things like that. So, there's that global effect. There's no direct effect [on individual physicians].

—physician, large multispecialty practice with 75 percent of revenue from capitation and shared savings contracts

However, once practices became financially successful under shared savings programs, some distributed their earnings to individual physicians based on each physician's productivity (as measured by RVUs or FFS revenues). As one puzzled respondent explained,

I'd say overall all the groups figured out eventually . . . that they would do some performance-based distribution of surplus or quality dollars [to individual physicians] and that a disproportionate share went to primary care because so many of the quality measures were in their hands . . . but sometimes for the [shared savings bonus,] some of them used the cheap way out: [distributing the bonus] as proportional to [FFS] revenue, which is reinforcing the wrong thing. . . . I mean, if you're trying to try a different model, why reinforce the old one?

—leader, health plan

Practical and Ethical Considerations Underlie Some Practice Leaders' Reluctance to Apply Financial Incentives for Cost Containment to Individual Physicians

Practice leaders' explanations for why they chose not to apply cost-containment financial incentives to individual physicians fell into two general categories. First, there were practical considerations: Adjusting for case mix and accounting for random variation in costs could be quite challenging. Second, several leaders and frontline physicians alike expressed ethical concerns about constructing financial incentives based on total costs of care because such incentives would not necessarily distinguish between better efficiency (i.e., eliminating unnecessary care) and stinting on care that actually was necessary. Such ethical concerns were broadly expressed by respondents from practices of varying size and specialties, though more frequently by hospital-owned practices. The following respondent explained both concerns:

This is the tension with all these incentives: . . . Do you make them individual or do you make them departmental or a blend of the two? What doctors always say . . . when they get their [cost] variation reports is, "I'm different. I'm special." There's always outliers . . . and that was my reaction too when I first started thinking about these things. But that's part of the reason it becomes very hard to bring [cost measures] back to their individual [compensation]. And I also think it creates an ethical tension that probably is not appropriate because what you don't want to do is put that individual physician in the position of making choices about [a] patient that are not in [the] patient's best interest because [the physician has] financial incentives to do so.

—leader, large multispecialty practice with 20 percent of revenue from capitation, shared savings, and PFP programs

Practices Applied Simplified Financial Incentives Linked to Quality of Care by Individual Physicians

Unlike how they handled incentives to contain the costs of care, some practices did transmit financial incentives linked to quality of care to individual physicians. Respondents representing a variety of practice sizes, specialties, and ownership structure and in most study markets noted this. For many practices, the range and multiplicity of quality incentives received from their payers was too great to be actionable for individual physicians, so the practice simplified the quality targets before transmitting quality-based financial incentives to physicians. In this example, by combining similar measures, one organization narrowed the 110 quality measures received from payers down to a somewhat more manageable set of 50 measures for primary care physicians:

> The way we've tried to deal with [having 110 quality measures] is we've tried to say to our docs: "Forget about the age differences in diabetes. All we want you to do is treat all your diabetics, no matter how old they are, the same way. Here are the five things we want you to do for them; and forget about the fact that, in [payment program X], if your cholesterol is high, it counts if you have a plan to lower it, whereas in [payment program Y], it doesn't. We want everybody to get the [low-density lipoprotein] actually the way it should be, under 100; and we ask that you be prudent, so if it's a critically ill 80-year-old or 50-year-old who's going to die of a cancer, I don't care that [that patient is] diabetic. Be rational about it." So we try to kind of teach people. . . . We come up with a basic principle and then we try to teach to that. So our docs aren't really looking at 110 measures. They may be looking at 50.
>
> —leader, large IPA with exposure to multiple capitation, shared savings, and
> PFP programs

To avoid overwhelming physicians, some practices chose explicitly to exclude certain quality measures entirely from individual physicians' financial incentives when these measures were too far afield from the bulk of PFP targets applied by multiple payers. For this practice, the risk of losing an incentive on one measure was preferable to the risk of overwhelming physicians and undermining performance improvement on all measures:

> [Performance measures are] 80 percent aligned [across payers] and about 20 percent not. That 20 percent causes all sorts of chaos. . . . So although we have all these external requirements for diabetes and hypertension and whatnot, inside of [our] system, we've taken all of these and we've rationalized them into one slate of measures that overlap as much as possible. . . . [But] sometimes there are one or two [external] targets that are still outside of [the internal slate of measures.] So we can meet the internal targets and still lose. And that's the risk at hand, but there's no real way around it without creating absolute chaos.
>
> —leader, large multispecialty practice with 20 percent of revenue from capitation, shared
> savings, and PFP programs

In Some Shared Savings and Capitation Models, Physicians Received Personal Financial Incentives for Specific Documentation Tasks

Participants in some shared savings and capitation programs reported fee for documentation as a new type of financial incentive to individual physicians. As one respondent explained, one

ACO sought to encourage thorough documentation of patients' diagnoses by applying such an incentive, noting that more-thorough diagnostic documentation could affect the hierarchical condition category mix for the ACO's patients:

> [The ACO] wants all the physicians to do a couple things—all the primary care physicians, they do [a diagnostic visit] similar to a Medicare Wellness Visit . . . and then they also have this document that they want the physicians to fill out themselves and sign that these are the diagnoses. . . . They incentivize it very heavily, financially. They have metrics that say, "If you do this many [diagnostic visits and documents] by the end of June, you get another little bonus. . . ." So if you get all the bonuses, it's at least three times what you would normally make in a given office visit. . . . What they want you to do is assess the patient's problems. Are you familiar with what [a hierarchical condition category] is? . . . It's the only time Medicare pays you just to get in there and clean up your charts.
>
> —physician, small primary care practice participating in a Medicare ACO program

We note that no interviewee in the study reported receiving any kind of incentive to misrepresent patients' health conditions. Instead, fee-for-documentation incentives were described as encouraging a thorough capture of diagnoses that truly were present but that might otherwise escape documentation because of the time and effort inherent in performing such documentation.

Nonfinancial Incentives and Other Interventions Applied to Physicians

When individual physician compensation was shielded from the financial incentives received by practices through alternative payment models, practices frequently described applying nonfinancial incentives and interventions to physicians instead. These incentives and interventions took a variety of forms, including performance feedback (with or without comparison to peer physicians), one-on-one management, physician education, institution of new care protocols, and selective retention of physicians in the practice.

Performance Feedback

Across study markets, practices of varying size, specialty, and ownership reported relying on performance feedback as a tool for motivating physicians to improve performance on measures of the quality and efficiency of care. This was most often reported by respondents in primary care and multispecialty practices.

Some practices, most commonly larger, multispecialty practices, even shared physicians' performance openly, seeking to appeal to inherent physicians' desire to be high performers. For example, in a subspecialty practice that was devising an episode-based payment program, the member physicians chose to couple a practice-level payment incentive with internal social pressure on individual physicians:

> [The incentive] will be as a group but split however many physicians are in it, so, if there's ten of us, we'll split it ten ways, and the idea there is . . . you specifically want to have it be where there's peer pressure for people to meet their performance goals . . . and having conversations, and if you need to, grab some help from others and sit down and talk to the

person. . . . "you can't just keep transfusing people at 8.5. . . . It hurts the performance measures and it's not good patient care."

> —subspecialist physician, small single-subspecialty practice

In another practice with substantial revenues derived from shared savings contracts, performance data were published even more openly:

> We are willing to . . . maintain the all-in group philosophy that there'll be enough pressure on the low-scoring people to up their scores because they know we publish the scores. . . . We publish those by name. It's on the Internet, . . . for every doctor. Anybody can see it. Patients can see it. . . . We believe that, if you publish the scores, people will be motivated to get better and elevate the department.

> —physician leader, large multispecialty practice

Other practices coupled performance reports with group discussions on how to improve:

> I don't just hand out the reports and leave it. I hand out the reports and then we discuss [best practices]. It kind of forces people to pay attention, and they are unblinded, so everyone sees everybody's numbers in terms of these reports. . . . With very few exceptions, people have ratcheted up their numbers.

> —physician leader, large multispecialty practice with shared savings tied to performance measures

Even when individual physician compensation was linked to performance on a given measure, feedback reporting could elicit a vigorous response—even among physicians who received bonus payments:

> Every doc here knows what the QI plan is, and most of them know what their targets are. . . . We allow an appeals process. If you think you got robbed on the measurement, we let people appeal. People appeal even when they get paid [a PFP bonus] just because they think their number was actually higher than the number that we recorded for them.

> —physician leader, large multispecialty practice

For some frontline physicians, however, a new emphasis on measuring their use of time seemed to encourage behavior that runs counter to the goal of producing more-efficient care. This was especially true when physicians were accountable for their "productivity" as measured by RVUs (which, as noted above, persisted as the dominant financial incentive in all markets, even in practices with significant capitation and shared savings exposure). As one respondent in a practice that had recently increased its share of its revenues from capitation and shared savings contracts explained,

> We used to not obsessively look at how much of our clinical time was utilized or how many encounters we had per week or, "Should I bill for this visit or not?" And now that [time utilization is] being measured, and they're trying to hold us more accountable for our time; I think there is a tendency to do the wrong thing, which is to churn patients, to say, "Well,

if they want me to fill my schedule up and they're going to penalize me if I have too much free time, I could call this patient with his lab in two weeks—[but the incentive is to] bring him back.

—subspecialist physician, large multispecialty practice

Changes to Care Protocols

Multiple practices and market observers reported that instituting standardized care protocols was a common response to episode-based payments. As with capitation and shared savings, no practice in our sample transmitted episode-based financial incentives to individual physicians directly (i.e., allowing some physicians in the practice to receive bonuses and others to be penalized under episode-based payment). Instead, practice leaders employed default order sets, education, and other nonfinancial tools to encourage physicians to adhere to standardized care protocols. These strategies were most frequently reported in larger practices, multispecialty practices, and hospital-owned practices. None of the surgical subspecialty practices in our sample reported using such approaches.

As one respondent in a practice receiving episode-based payments for CHF admissions explained, a carefully designed CHF order set coupled with encouragement to use the order set was well-received by other physicians:

One of the things that we struggled with was a lot of patients with CHF [being] admitted initially with shortness of breath, so [patients] weren't getting that initial CHF order set, right? So those patients, for us, were falling through the cracks, and so it took some education of physicians to say, "You know, if your patient admits with shortness of breath, always consider CHF . . . even if you're not diagnosing them with CHF as an admitting diagnosis, that doesn't mean that you can't use the CHF order set to make sure that the patient doesn't get behind in [his or her] care." . . . Our docs want to do the right thing. They want to take care of their patients in the most evidence-based way. We definitely didn't have any belligerence on their part at all.

—physician, small single-subspecialty practice

In some cases, the act of designing a care protocol caused physicians to reexamine their longstanding care patterns, identifying low-hanging fruit for cost containment under episode-based payments. For example, in one practice, substantial savings were achieved by simply realizing that previous default postoperative destinations were unnecessarily expensive, and changing these defaults was a key intervention:

[The surgeons] actually have moved the needle on where people are getting their care after discharge. It used to be 80 percent of their [postoperative] care went to [skilled-nursing facilities] or rehab. And now close to 80 percent of the people go home. . . . They've been engaged also in this kind of "prehab," rehabilitation ahead of time before the surgery, etc. [The key step] was probably putting information in front of the surgeons, where they kind of realized that they never [noticed before] that so many people were just automatically going to these high-cost [postoperative facilities].

—leader, large multispecialty practice

Similarly, standardizing the choice of medical devices was another successful strategy, especially relative to the lack of standardization that existed previously:

> I think [subspecialists are] going to have to agree to more-structured standardization. I mean, you might have a group of [orthopedists] today, . . . Each one of the doctors in the practice could be using a different hip replacement from a different vendor, different manufacturer with widely variant costs. And so those kinds of things are going to have to change. . . . You're going to see more standardization of things, more standardization in prescribing patterns. . . . We're already starting to see it a little bit with the episode payments, that providers are starting to make changes in their practice.
>
> —leader, health plan

Selective Retention of Physicians

Larger practices that received capitation or shared savings payments reported using selective recruiting and retention as a cost-containment tool. Termination of physicians from the practice was described as a last option, applied only after performance feedback and education had failed to produce desired changes.

For example, selective retention of physicians was illustrated in a practice with greater than 50 percent of revenue at risk via capitation and shared savings contracts but—like the other practices in our sample—no financial incentives for cost containment for individual physicians. Instead, the practice applied management techniques to physicians who were high-cost outliers and, in certain cases, terminated recalcitrant physicians:

> People generally respond well to management, particularly people who are . . . otherwise good contributing members to your team. Most people don't want to do poorly. . . . Then there are others . . . who just deny and accuse and pass the buck—and you know they're not going to get better. Those people might not be the best member on your team in the future. . . . So, there's been a few terminations since I've been here in the [specialty] clinic and in other surgical specialties and medical specialties. . . . We've been more aggressive at attacking those outliers or the past year or two than we had previously.
>
> —physician leader, large multispecialty practice

Similarly, a single-specialty practice in which contact capitation accounted for the vast majority of revenue prioritized "like-mindedness" in recruiting its physicians. Within the practice, individual physicians then received salaries plus bonuses for productivity (based on RVUs) and adherence to evidence-based practices, but no financial incentives for cost control:

> We knew that the track we were on was the right one, and that was to capitate for large patient volumes. That way you can control the cost; you can control the quality. And if you're willing to manage them appropriately, then you can minimize the risk. So we practiced evidence-based medicine, [and] we hire like-minded physicians who want to be part of that. Actually, in our job advertisements, that's one of the main things we focus on, and when I get most candidates, that's what they really like—they like the evidence-based practice. So the physicians here are employees, and they all practice the same brand of medicine.
>
> —administrative leader, medium-sized single-subspecialty practice

Some practice leaders noted generational differences in cohorts of physicians who trained under different prevailing payment arrangements. For example, physicians who established their practice patterns when capitation was common (e.g., in the 1990s) were different from those who came of age when FFS predominated (e.g., in the mid-2000s). This respondent described the current situation, in which practices had historically hired physicians who could generate large revenues under FFS, though recent pendulum swings to capitation and shared savings resulted in a mismatch between physician proclivities and these alternative payment programs:

> When you're in [a] fee-for-service model, [whom] do you hire? You hire [subspecialists] who are highly productive, and they're not necessarily the people who are also communicating with their colleagues or saying [to primary care physicians], "Don't send me back that patient. You got it. I'm going to hand off back to you. They're stable now." . . . So we ended up hiring a lot of highly productive people, and we also paid them on [an] RVU-based model. [But] as a corporation, we're not paid on units [anymore]; we're paid on total value. . . . [We] need a whole generation to retire, but we [also] need a new generation to understand the value model.

> —leader, large multispecialty practice

Changes in Total Physician Compensation

Practices in all six of the markets in our study reported declining or stagnant FFS payment rates, with the exception of the significant increases in Medicaid payment rates to primary care physicians in 2013 and 2014 under the ACA. Against this background, the effects of alternative payment models were generally neutral (especially in new episode-based payment programs, which, for some practices, accounted for "such an infinitesimal, small amount of money that it didn't amount to much") to positive with regard to the aggregate amount of physician compensation. For example, in an ACO that had received a shared savings bonus in the previous year, physicians received significantly more total compensation than they would have received under FFS:

> In the [shared savings program], we see that doctors are getting paid somewhere between 115 percent and 130 percent of what they would be paid by [FFS] alone. So, it's a pretty good deal. . . . Once they saw [that] the bonus was real, they paid attention.

> —leader, large multispecialty practice

Aspirational Payment Models

Some physicians in our sample, especially those in smaller practices with limited exposure to alternative payment models, expressed strong desires to participate in payment models other than FFS. In general, these physicians hoped that these alternative payment models would produce better alignment between what they should do (i.e., how they should optimally allocate their effort to produce efficient, high-quality patient care) and what they were paid to do. Put another way, there appeared to be an underlying desire to eliminate the implicit cross-subsidy between highly paid activities and more–poorly paid activities that were possibly more important for patient care.

For example, one surgeon who reported spending significant time improving patient care protocols at a local hospital, with minimal compensation for these efforts under FFS, described episode-based payments as a way of sharing in the benefits that he was creating by engaging in these activities, rather than performing an extra surgery (which was much more highly compensated):

> If there's stuff I could do to make . . . my patient experience, outcome, satisfaction, and safety better, fantastic. I'm willing to do some of that for free, but . . . if I'm going to be taking hours out of my business day to be doing that . . . How about a little something for the effort?
>
> —physician, small single-subspecialty practice

Comparison Between Current Findings and Previously Published Research

Prior literature indicates that practice participation in capitated-payment models is associated with a greater likelihood of salary-based, rather than productivity-based, compensation arrangements for individual physicians (Robinson, Shortell, Li, et al., 2004; Robinson, Casalino, et al., 2009). In our sample, however, even "salaried" physicians in practices that received significant shares of their revenues through global capitation or shared savings models still had productivity incentives at the margin (e.g., through RVU-based bonuses). Our finding is consistent with recently published research reporting that physician salaries are frequently adjusted for productivity in "leading health systems" taking global capitation and participating in ACO demonstrations (Khullar et al., 2014).

CHAPTER TEN

Physician Work and Professional Satisfaction

Overview of Findings

In our sample, alternative payment models had not changed substantially how physicians delivered face-to-face patient care. However, increases in nonclinical work were a source of discontent. Though some physicians recognized the value of the added documentation requirements in certain instances (e.g., for identifying gaps in care), many physicians in our sample reported expansion of nonclinical work that they perceived to be irrelevant to patient care (e.g., duplicating and reporting data already contained in patients' medical records to fulfill contractual obligations). In addition, as detailed in Chapter Six, physicians in practices participating in global capitation or shared savings payment models reported new clinical activities stemming from collaboration between primary care physicians and subspecialist physicians (e.g., generating joint treatment plans for complex patients).

Physicians perceived that, by and large, most alternative payment models had increased both the quantity and the intensity of physician work. The quantity was driven by a need to maintain or expand patient volumes, either as part of certain payment models, such as capitation, or as a defense strategy against potential downside risk from alternative payment models. The increased intensity resulted from ongoing pressure for physicians to practice at the "top of license," which was noted to be a potential source of burnout because lower-intensity patients might actually be an important source of respite for busy physicians.

The effects that changing payment models have had on the levels of work-related satisfaction among physicians in practice leadership positions have been somewhat different from those for physicians not in leadership roles. Most physician leaders were optimistic and enthusiastic about alternative payment models; most physicians not in leadership roles expressed at least some level of apprehension, particularly with regard to the documentation requirements of new payment models. Overall, physicians seemed to believe that major change in payment methods will continue and acknowledged that change is needed and that some changes are useful. Nevertheless, their attitude was one of resignation, rather than enthusiasm, because their day-to-day work life had become more difficult and included burdens that they believed would not improve patient care.

Detailed Findings

Work Content

Overall, most physicians reported little impact from recent payment and organizational changes on how they spend their clinical time when face to face with patients. This was noted by respondents in all markets, in practices of varying size, specialty, and ownership structure. In fact, face-to-face clinical work was predominantly perceived to be a positive aspect of physician work, with respondents noting that direct patient care is what physicians are trained to do and, by and large, what they like to do. In addition, some respondents noted that alternative payment models supported physicians' performance of patient care activities other than face-to-face care, which many had been doing already, but without payment under FFS. This respondent in a practice that had recently implemented a medical home model reported,

> [The physicians are] primarily doing the same level of patient care, and that's one of the things that has made these patient-centered medical home metrics easy for us: . . . that I have good docs and they practice good-quality care anyway. . . . Now we're getting paid for a lot of the stuff that we've always done, where we did recall and we do phone call care and we do make sure [patients are] up to date on their immunizations and we do help them with their referrals and schedule with specialists and everything and do have really [to] follow up with our patients anyway.
>
> —practice administrator, small primary care practice

Subspecialists reported less impact of alternative payment models on their work, as described by this respondent whose practice participated in a PFP program:

> It's not a whole lot different from our point of view. . . . It's a really tiny part of our world. . . . If you ask me what are our [PFP program] measures, I probably couldn't tell you. I mean I know them. . . . If someone showed them to me, I'd go, "Yeah, yeah, yeah." . . . but it's really not a big part of our world. . . . It really doesn't influence us. We come in; we do our job; we go home. Whether or not we're making [the payer] happy is a bit irrelevant to us.
>
> —physician, small single–medical subspecialty practice

Other physician leaders did report that alternative payment models had prompted the development of initiatives that might lead to changes in the content of physicians' clinical work and that such changes could be difficult. This respondent in a practice participating in PFP, shared savings, and medical home payment models described changes targeted at achieving greater efficiency in the delivery of patient care:

> No doctor likes to change. There are some early adopters; there are some middle adopters; there's some late adopters. Docs are no different in that regard, and that's what we're facing. But overall, people recognize the need to change and they are moving along. . . .
>
> —physician leader, large multispecialty practice

Work Quantity and Intensity
Physicians in Nearly All Alternative Payment Models Are Encouraged to Increase Both the Quantity and Intensity of Work

Respondents in nearly all markets, at practices of varying sizes, ownership models, and specialties, described a variety of different levers used by different alternative payment models, such as incentives for physicians to practice at the top of license, pressures to increase patient volume, both as part of payment models, such as capitation, and in an effort to maintain FFS income while transitioning to alternative payment models. This respondent shared the tensions and workload shifts that occur in a market in which most primary care physicians are capitated for primary care services (and subspecialists are not):

> The disturbing thing is that, as people get pressed for time, primary care doctors have less and less interest in doing the basic stuff. . . . In the good old days, [primary care physicians] would actually take an interest in headaches and . . . do some stuff before they said, "Oh, well, go see a neurologist." But, under this system, when primary care is paid a set fee for, let's say, 2,000 patients per month, they get a check in the mail every month for those 2,000 patients, and the only [incentive] is to do the least amount of work that they possibly can, which involves basically sending somebody to a specialist at the drop of a hat because any work they do is . . . included in their capitation payment.

> —physician, small single-subspecialty practice

Although practicing at the top of license is often promoted as a positive development in achieving greater efficiencies in the provision of health care, another respondent also reported that this greater level of intensity could be unsustainable:

> There's a lot of burnout in primary care. It's a really hard job, and we're trying to figure that out to keep good people practicing. Working at top of license, you know, you can look at it like, "So, why are you seeing this sore throat when you could be seeing a, you know, congestive heart failure and letting your nurse practitioner see your sore throat?" You know, it's that sore throat that kind of gives you a breather sometimes during the day. So, it's a two-edged sword. . . .

> —physician, large multispecialty practice

Professional Satisfaction
Physicians in Leadership Positions

Physicians in leadership positions were enthusiastic about new opportunities to improve patient care provided by alternative payment methods. This was noted most frequently by small primary care and medical subspecialty practices of varying ownership structures throughout our study markets.

Many physician leaders were able to examine the effect of alternative payment models from a broad perspective, understanding that their ultimate goal was to improve the delivery of health care while providing cost savings and high quality. This respondent was enthused by his work and his role in making care better:

> I think we're seeing really some major changes coming about in how we're going to deliver. And I think the dictums you read on accessibility to care, patient experience in that care, service quality, however you want to measure that, the clinical quality parameters, metrics, I'm all for it. And that's fine. . . . So take a group like ours; we're working on quality parameters and trying to focus on certain things, [such as] quality parameters . . . Already I'm seeing the practice beginning to think about things. . . . There's just so much opportunity for us to improve things. I wish I had 30 more years to be part of it.
>
> —physician leader, medium-sized single-subspecialty practice

Similarly, another respondent in a group that has engaged in risk contracting for many years expressed great enthusiasm for making risk contracting more widespread:

> As we look forward to value-based payments, we couldn't be more excited. It speaks to all of our strengths. . . . There's enough money in the entire system here such that, if we can now migrate away from incentives that incent providers economically based upon how much of something they do . . . but we can now focus them more on saying, . . . "You're achieving these quality scores; you're achieving this kind of quality and this kind of patient satisfaction . . . and if you're doing it for less, then there's no reason why you should not benefit from that." . . . I absolutely love that.
>
> —physician leader, medium-sized single-subspecialty practice

Physicians Not in Leadership Roles

Physicians not in leadership roles reported significant discontent, largely resulting from the increased burdens of documentation required in alternative payment models. In theory, primary care physicians should benefit from payment methods that emphasize value and population health. These goals are consonant with the objectives and skill sets of primary care, should put primary care physicians in important roles within medical groups, and should, by increasing the demand for primary care, lead to higher incomes for primary care physicians. However, respondents in our study were more likely to report that, in particular, the reporting requirements of alternative payment models had negatively affected their lives. This respondent, whose practice participated in capitation, FFS, PFP, and medical home payment models, reported,

> I think that there's a decrease in professional satisfaction because it's become more of a metric-driven entity than an art, in terms of your day-to-day [clinical practice], and I think a decrease in satisfaction. . . . It is particularly acute in primary care.
>
> —physician, large multispecialty practice

Even when physicians not in leadership roles reported having faith in the potential benefits of alternative payment models, the pressures of required documentation were a significant source of unhappiness. For physicians in all specialties and practice sizes, it could be difficult to separate new documentation requirements stemming from alternative payment models from the changes in documentation activities caused by adopting EHRs. This respondent participating in a shared savings program recounted,

> The [shared savings program], for us, is a no-brainer. . . . My own feeling is it's doing good medicine. So that is a win-win for us. It's what the electronic medical records [require] that is the lose-lose for us. Yes, they can read my writing now, but it's added hours to every day and it's taken up all the weekends, so it's really destroyed quality of life and, for instance, my son, who graduated from medical school [a] couple of years ago, looked at what I'm doing and he said, "Dad, you're nuts. You have no life." He went into radiology. . . . Who would want to spend 12 hours a day and most of the weekend massaging the record?
>
> —physician, small primary care practice

Despite misgivings and increased burdens on physician practices, some physicians not in leadership roles expressed optimism about the promise of alternative payment models. This respondent, whose practice participates in shared savings, felt rejuvenated by the potential of alternative payment models to increasingly align the incentives in health care for the better:

> I see, finally, that the payment is aligning with the good of the patient and the severity of illness, which has not quite been the case before. So I think more of that needs to happen, and I think we need to look at the cost of taking care of a population. And I hope that happens.
>
> —physician, small primary care practice

Another respondent expressed willingness, at least for the time being, to make the trade-off between, on the one hand, the inconvenience and increased work required to document requirements of alternative payment models in an EHR and, on the other hand, better care for patients:

> I think it's helpful for patients, the guidelines, to look at them, when they're due for a mammogram . . . if they're due for colonoscopy. . . . so that's important that they give us those guidelines to look at. . . . Working with the computer when you're working with a patient, it's a lot of work . . . getting everything done that you're supposed to get done. So you're supposed to look at the guidelines on every patient and check the things that are due. . . . It's just a lot of work. But I mean, it's helpful for the patient because it's preventative medicine.
>
> —physician, large multispecialty practice

Physician Leadership

Interviewees in all markets and in multiple roles, representing hospitals, health plans, medical societies, and larger physician practices, described physician leaders as being critical to gaining buy-in from other physicians in the practice for participation in alternative payment models. Fewer respondents in small practices mentioned physician leadership as a specific key to success, perhaps because leadership was defined less formally in such practices.

Some organizations funded leadership positions for physicians, who were expected to serve as liaisons between administrative leadership and the other physicians:

> I think you really have to have physician leadership. It has to be driven by physicians, and we have a medical director [whose] full-time job is to cultivate these relationships. . . . He is meeting with the physicians because, if you don't have the physicians as leaders at the table, the ACO will not be successful. You've got to have dedicated physician leadership in order for these things to work well and to work effectively because it's not about just how we pay them; it's changing the way care is delivered, and the only people [who] can do that are those [who] are delivering the care.

> —leader, health plan

Similarly, this respondent shared the differences between the physician leadership needs in old models of care and those required by alternative payment models:

> In the old model, which was managed care 1.0, where it was about rationing, you didn't need medical judgment in order to say, "No, you can't do that." In an environment in which you're trying to develop the most appropriate care, the care that will provide the best result at the lowest possible cost, you can't do that without physician leadership. It's not possible. . . .

> —leader, hospital

Physician Leaders Require a Specific Set of Skills for Which Few Physicians Are Trained
Other respondents noted that physician leaders need specific skills and that the skills acquired by being physician leaders under existing payment models might not necessarily translate into skills that are appropriate for leading an organization participating in alternative payment models:

> Some of [the missing leadership skill set] was just basics, like, how do you run a meeting effectively? [During the managed care era of the 1990s,] a lot of docs who were medical directors in IPAs or PHOs were, in some sense, the poor sucker who was the last man standing when everyone took a step back. . . . Mostly it was being trotted out for a contract negotiation. . . . so many of them lacked a lot of basics. . . . Another key piece was, how do you manage a group of physicians or, better yet, lead a group of physicians without getting caught up in the distractions of someone [who] wants to sabotage the direction or someone who likes to hear themselves talk . . . and keep guiding them in a productive direction? . . . Another key piece was around financials. Many of them hadn't had to deal with balance sheets, and how do you do accounting and how do you know whether you're succeeding or not succeeding?

> —physician, large multispecialty practice

Unfortunately, respondents also noted that it is challenging to identify physicians with both the skills and the interest to serve in leadership positions:

> The biggest challenge that I have as the chief executive of our integrated delivery system is getting a sufficient number of physicians willing to step up to lead the care processes. We need physician leadership badly. Designing the systems, understanding the variation, reducing the variation, understanding the per member per month, financial management elements of this. . . . that's probably the most important element to success of this entire enterprise going forward. . . . You really need to get them in there and working and give them sufficient time in order to do so. So, that's a real challenge. It can't be just one or two guys. It's got to be a whole culture.
>
> —leader, hospital

Other Forms of Physician Engagement

The creation and implementation of alternative payment models provides many opportunities for physician engagement, some of which could involve relatively minimal effort. Physician engagement opportunities were discussed by all types of respondents, including hospitals, health plans, medical societies, MGMA chapters, and practices of all sizes, specialties, and ownership, throughout our study markets.

To broaden the scope of physician engagement, some practices (particularly medium-sized and large practices) created multiple opportunities for involvement:

> Why that's important is, if you look at all of those committees plus the board, there's somewhere [around] 50 physicians out of the 500 [in the IPA.] So that means that 10 percent of the IPA is very involved in what we're doing.
>
> —physician leader, IPA

Physician engagement also included simply reviewing and reacting to data or other feedback provided by practices as part of alternative payment models. However, the extent of such engagement was variable:

> One of the goals of the clinically integrated network is to get physicians access to their data benchmarked against the quality measures. . . . Those [who] are using it are beginning to start looking at things, drill into the data, question what's going on. . . . That's a 12- to 18-month transformation. . . . Ten percent really grab a hold of that and go with it. You know, 80 percent will kind of go along after a while, and 10 percent will never look at it. They'll be able to start looking at their own data benchmarked and be able to do that any time they want to. And that's on all their patients. We upload every bit of their diagnostic data any time they send it out to the insurance companies.
>
> —leader, hospital

Finally, in the face of a paucity of quality measures in use for subspecialist physicians, some groups have found ways to engage subspecialists in transforming health care as part of participation in some alternative payment models:

> That's a great question [about quality measures for specialists] and one which we still struggle with. When we give out surplus . . . we take 15 percent of the surplus and we put it towards quality metrics. The 15 percent on the quality side is that our specialists are required to do a quality project. . . . About 60 percent of our specialists actually do quality improvement projects and get the money.

> —physician leader, IPA

Comparison Between Current Findings and Previously Published Research

Previous research has indicated that some physicians have "expressed significant anger about and suspicion of financial incentives for quality" (Teleki et al., 2006, p. 371), which is consistent with our finding that some physicians, especially those not in leadership roles, reported that the PFP programs in which they participated encourage them to invest additional time in documenting care rather than providing care.

With regard to physician satisfaction, in a survey of primary care physicians, 30 percent of respondents reportedly "viewed extrinsic pressures to standardize care as contrary to their clinical judgment," and that perception was associated with a higher likelihood of job dissatisfaction (Waddimba et al., 2013). This is consistent with findings from our study, in which respondents expressed displeasure when they perceived that bureaucratic processes were driving patient care. Findings from the current study also are concordant with our prior study on physician satisfaction, which found that physician professional satisfaction was lower under conditions of excessive time pressure and work intensity (Friedberg, Chen, et al., 2013).

Existing evidence also reports on the growing importance of physician leadership as mirrored in our study findings. In the National Survey of ACOs from October 2012 to May 2013, 51 percent of the respondent ACOs reported being physician-led, 33 percent jointly led with a hospital, and 3 percent hospital-led (V. Lewis, Colla, Carluzzo, et al., 2013). Further, in this survey, respondents in physician-led ACOs expressed more optimism about the ACO model's dissemination and potential to improve quality.

CHAPTER ELEVEN

Factors Limiting the Effectiveness of New Payment Models as Implemented

Overview of Findings

The implementation of new payment programs can uncover unanticipated problems that limit their effectiveness, at least temporarily. The physician practices in our sample described encountering a few key types of operational problems when participating in new payment programs. By taking steps to avoid or prepare for these stumbling points, designers and implementers of future payment programs might be able to enhance their likelihood of achieving program goals.

First, physicians and practice leaders participating in a variety of alternative payment models (any model other than FFS) described encountering errors in data integrity and timeliness, performance measure specification, and patient attribution. These payment models shared characteristics that might have made errors more likely: They were administratively more complex than FFS payment; some required payers to develop new measurement systems; and some were deployed for the first time quite quickly, without a "dress rehearsal" in which errors could be corrected before payments were on the line. Moreover, several physician practices reported experiences that led them to believe that some payers were waiting for physician practices to detect operational errors, rather than taking steps to ensure program integrity before making or withholding payments. Future participants in such models might consider such dress rehearsals or at least asking payers to design systems to detect and correct implementation errors, which might be inevitable even in the best of cases.

Second, physicians had a variety of concerns about the implementation of performance and risk-adjustment measures underlying PFP, shared savings, and capitation programs. Broadly speaking, these concerns stemmed from a sense that the multiplicity of measures within and across programs could distract physician practices from making the changes to patient care that were actually the ultimate goal of many payment programs.

Third, the influence of uncontrollable, game-changing events in shared savings and capitation programs (e.g., the introduction of very high-cost specialty drugs) sapped physician practices' enthusiasm for these payment models. Finally, some physicians reported that they could not understand exactly what behaviors were being encouraged or discouraged by certain performance-based payment programs—even after seeking clarification from payers. Although these physicians reported that the performance bonuses they received were welcome, an incentive that its target does not understand how to earn might not function as intended. Therefore, when necessary, investing in the understandability of incentive programs might enhance their effectiveness.

Detailed Findings

Errors in Payment Program Execution

Physicians and practice leaders from practices of all sizes, specialties, and ownership models and nearly all markets described experiences with errors in the execution of new alternative payment programs. In some cases, these errors resulted in nonpayment of earned bonuses; in others, they created an ongoing sense of uncertainty because performance feedback data were viewed as unreliable. In general, however, interviewees remained optimistic about the fundamental goals and designs of these new programs, despite these operational hiccups, and were willing to continue participation—provided that operational errors were corrected.

For example, one single-subspecialty practice participating in an episode-based payment program reported nonpayment of earned bonuses (for achieving lower-than-target costs of care per episode) because of two health plan operational errors: first, incomplete data capture, and second, an error in specification of a key quality measure. This practice had invested considerable resources in reengineering its approach to patient care and looked forward to eventually receiving its earned bonus payment to offset these costs:

> We remapped how we were going to take care of these patients. We wrote a new treatment plan, and we said we were going to get everyone back into the clinic and see them within one week after discharge. . . . And then, we went live, [and], for the most part, we've always fallen into the favorable category, that we should get some money back from the [health plan], but we haven't. . . . So, we figured something must be wrong and, oh, it took us forever, but we finally got through to [the health plan], and they said, "Oh, yeah . . . something is wrong." This was a year ago . . . but I'm still not certain if it's corrected. . . . I'm suspicious that it's not yet. But I'm challenged because it's hard for me to figure out if we've been on the mark all the time or not. It's been very, very difficult running it down.
>
> —subspecialist physician, small single-subspecialty practice

A small number of primary care practices in our study participated in multiple medical home programs, each with different rules for attributing patients. These attribution rules were critically important to each program because they identified the patients who served as the bases for per-patient per-month fees, performance measure calculation, and computation of shared savings. Therefore, errors in patient attribution could distort medical home–related payments in several ways. This respondent from a practice that examined its rosters of attributed patients explained,

> We've had some challenges with [the health plan] to get [it] to acknowledge that we don't see [some patients attributed to us]—I mean, we found deceased patients; we found patients who hadn't been here in five years, but they were still on the [health plan] records, and [the health plan] doesn't have a system in place to update [its] database of allocated members on a timely basis. . . .
>
> —leader, medium-sized primary care practice

Another respondent remarked more generally on how the complexity inherent in payment programs that rely on procedure and diagnosis coding to perform risk adjustment and generate quality data created opportunities for error at multiple steps in the process, both for clinicians and for payers:

> [Data are] all collected from the claim form that's entered. So as an organization or as a health care provider, CPT coding and diagnosis coding [are] very important because the health of your business . . . is really measured through all of that CPT coding. . . . You know, there's error on the provider side, if they don't enter it into the system. There's error with the [billing] system if it doesn't drop the claim properly. There's error in the translation of the claim to the [payment] system for whatever IPA or health plan or whatever is [accessing the data]. There's error in knowledge base of the person who's actually reading it or pulling it down and how it's interpreted. There's a lot of room for error.
>
> —physician, large primary care practice

Concerns About Performance Measure Implementation

In general, physicians and practice leaders in our sample agreed with the fundamental goals of performance measurement and liked the idea of being paid more (or at least not being paid less) when they provided better patient care. However, they cited multiple types of concerns about calculating these measures for the purpose of operationalizing alternative payment programs, ranging from PFP to shared savings to capitation. The concerns detailed in this section centered on whether, as measures made the transition from concept to implementation, their ability to truly assess the quality and efficiency of care (and thereby encourage desirable changes in patient care) was attenuated.

For example, interviewees from a variety of practice sizes, specialties, and ownership models across multiple markets described a cacophony of performance measures stemming from different payers and payment programs. Faced with having too many performance measures to mount a meaningful response, some described a sense of being encouraged to "win a game" rather than make fundamental changes to patient care. As one respondent in a practice participating in multiple shared savings and PFP programs explained,

> The PQRS [measures] don't line up particularly well with the meaningful-use ones and, you know, all sorts of other [measures.] It's like [having] 50 people shouting their priorities at you, and then trying to prioritize those into some semblance of order. . . . It does have this, sort of, feeling of "make-work" at some level. . . . You lose sight of [whether] this is really having true clinical impact or is this just, you know, like winning the video game? And that's what it starts to feel like after a while when you have a list of 50 things that you're chasing.
>
> —leader, large multispecialty practice

For some subspecialties in which few performance measures existed previously, physicians described the implementation of brand-new performance measures as part of their participation in new payment programs. In some cases, these physicians expressed concern about whether high or low performance on these measures truly reflected differences in patient care—as opposed to differences in case mix and random variation in patient needs. This respondent, who had received a bonus in one such PFP program, explained how doubts about the measure created a perception that bonus payments were distributed arbitrarily:

> [The performance measure] was a stupid one to do: the rate at which you order advanced radiology images. I'm not sure what the right number is for a surgeon to order [magnetic resonance imaging scans] and [computed tomography scans], but it's more than zero, right? And it's very much dependent on your practice. . . . And one of the things I [told the health plan was], "I don't know why you guys are using this as a metric for me because I can tell you, within my own given practice, it's going to be wildly variable." . . . Except I got a bonus check. And other specialists didn't. . . . Yeah, it was like the tooth fairy. I woke up, and there was check under my pillow.
>
> —physician, small single-subspecialty practice

Physicians across all markets perceived that success in performance measurement was sometimes driven by coding practices rather than true differences in patient care, particularly when payments under certain capitation and shared savings programs relied on coding-based risk adjustment. As one respondent in a practice that was part of an ACO (and subject to shared savings incentives) had learned over time, choosing specific diagnostic codes and leaving no diagnosis uncoded were encouraged:

> So it's a little bit of a game. You could be depressed, 311, or you could be depressed, 296. . . . One's risk adjusted, and the other one is not. . . . So now that I'm going to get credit, I'm definitely going to pick [the diagnostic code that triggers risk adjustment]. And risk-adjusted depression in remission counts. . . . A diabetic patient you can just go to town on. Diabetes with renal problems, diabetes with endocrine problems, diabetes with obesity—that's everyone—diabetes with cardiovascular, with ophthalmology, with neurology problems. . . .This creating of the [risk-adjustment] score, you know, encourages people to code better and code more.
>
> —physician, small primary care practice within an ACO

Finally, in some cases, physicians reported that the performance measures included in new payment programs set too low a bar for improvement, especially when measures seemed to be selected to give the impression of high performance without requiring any changes in patient care. For some physicians who were excited about making major changes to their practices, starting with such measures created a sense of impatience for more-meaningful performance measurement. As one respondent in a newly forming ACO explained,

> Some of it feels a little bit canned. I mean, it's really not physician led. It's really consultant led. . . . We want to have quality measures . . . but they're mostly stuff we're already doing . . . and in my opinion, they don't really drive quality of care like they should. . . . That doesn't feel very [meaningful. However,] for the first time in my [medical career], I have to say we are on the right track. Finally, we're saying, "Let us measure outcomes and let us make sure that we're doing the right thing for patients all the time." . . . But what we currently have set up for measures is not going to change much, and we hope that rapidly [we]

replace them with [measures] that are little more challenging and maybe things that actually do make more of a difference.

—physician, small single-subspecialty practice

Uncontrollable Factors in Risk Contracts

Unanticipated events that physician practices perceived as being beyond their control were described as threats to continued participation in certain alternative payment models—especially shared savings and capitation models that incentivized global cost containment. Such concerns were noted by leaders of large practices, especially those engaged in global capitation or shared savings contracts with downside financial risk. As one leader of a large practice with multiple shared savings contracts explained, the recent emergence of very high-cost specialty pharmacy drugs overwhelmed the practice's efforts to control total costs of care:

> Things like this specialty pharmacy undercut all of the efforts. I mean, if we're going to be sabotaged by drug pricing that we don't control, then why bother, right? There's no motivation for us to take any risk at all. . . . We're not insurance companies. We don't have experience in that. So medical management, sure, we can work on that, but we can't be held hostage to events that are out of our control. . . . I think ideally you would just carve [specialty pharmacy] out completely. Because . . . if you want to grow momentum [in favor of shared savings payment models], you have to show people that you are succeeding in it. So when all of a sudden . . . our [cost] trend is just garbage and we've been working so hard at it, that's very discouraging.

> —physician leader, large multispecialty practice

Similarly, multiple interviewees in other practices engaged in risk-based payment models (capitation, shared savings, and episode-based payment) expressed a desire for reinsurance against uncontrollable, extremely high-cost events, or exclusion of such costs from their spending targets.

Understandability of Incentives

In some alternative payment programs, particularly those that featured new performance measures or combinations of performance measures for physicians, some physicians reported being unable to understand what they were being incentivized to do—i.e., they did not know (and, in some cases, could not figure out, despite making considerable efforts) how to modify their patient care to achieve better performance. Even among physicians who did well under new performance measures, some reported lacking a clear idea of how to increase their likelihood of receiving another bonus in the future. This confusion was reported most often by small primary care or single-subspecialty practices and was not reported by respondents in any large multispecialty practices in this study (perhaps because large practices acted as intermediaries that selectively transmitted understandable incentives to individual physicians).

As one surgeon who received a performance bonus explained,

> [The health plan] asked me if could I help other [doctors] achieve the same [performance] bonus. [But] I couldn't tell what to tell them to do. . . . We'd been on the phone for almost

an hour; I couldn't understand their formulas. I couldn't understand the factors that played into it. [So] I still couldn't tell people, "You ought to do more of this and less of that."

—physician, small single-subspecialty practice

Comparison Between Current Findings and Previously Published Research

We found that many physicians and practice leaders had concerns about the implementation of some quality measures (especially when improving performance seemed to depend more on changing documentation than on changing clinical care), and these concerns were reported as limiting the effectiveness of alternative payment models that depend on such measures. These findings are concordant with prior literature describing physicians' concerns that PFP might reward improved documentation rather than true improvements in care (Petersen et al., 2006; Berenson and Kaye, 2013; Berenson, Pronovost, and Krumholz, 2013; Eijkenaar et al., 2013).

For some alternative payment models, our findings indicate that their widespread diffusion might be limited by their complexity, which creates opportunities for operational errors and impairs physicians' ability to understand exactly what changes in clinical care are being encouraged. Prior research describing two attempts to implement new episode-based, bundled payment programs also found barriers that likely stemmed, in part, from complexity of these payment models (Hussey, Ridgely, and Rosenthal, 2011; Ridgely et al., 2014).

CHAPTER TWELVE

Conclusions

Nearly all physicians, physician practice leaders, and market observers who participated in this project described multiple simultaneous changes in payment programs and regulations. Most interviewees therefore described how interactions between these simultaneous changes, rather than the introduction of a given specific alternative payment model, affected physicians and physician practices. Some interactions were synergistic, such as when EHRs had the potential to enable physician practices to achieve PFP targets, while others were antagonistic, such as conflicting incentives and measures from different payers.

Throughout the study, with the exception of independent solo practitioners, we found that physician practices played important roles as intermediaries and buffers between changes in the health care marketplace (including but not limited to alternative payment models) and individual practicing physicians. In some instances, practices magnified the effects of alternative payment models on physicians' approaches to patient care by, for example, making substantial investments in new care pathways to enable successful performance in episode-based payment programs, even when such programs accounted for a negligible percentage of practice revenues. In other instances, practices shielded their physicians completely from specific aspects of alternative payment models—for example, when practice leaders made conscious decisions to ignore certain PFP measures to give their physicians a manageable array of targets for improvement. Physician practices also described translating external financial incentives from health plans into nonfinancial incentives for individual physicians within the practice; this translation was nearly universal for financial incentives to contain the costs of care.

Practice leaders expressed considerable uncertainty about best strategies for responding to the combinations of alternative payment models that they faced, and these uncertainties were compounded by doubts about the future. Would payment models that are currently little more than novelties (e.g., episode-based payment programs) become commonplace, thus rewarding disproportionate efforts to excel in early programs? Will risk-based payment models that currently seem ascendant (e.g., ACOs and shared savings) persist for several more years, or will the pendulum swing back to FFS?

Guided by practical limits on available capital and how much change their physicians can absorb quickly (especially when "change" amounted to "more work for each physician"), practice leaders tended to proceed cautiously, prioritizing areas in which multiple payment incentives overlapped with each other and with practices' internal priorities. For some smaller, independent practices, merging with larger practices or hospitals was an attractive option for accessing the capital necessary to succeed in alternative payment models, complying with new regulations (such as meaningful use), and enhancing their ability to control what alternative payment models they faced and how these would affect their physicians.

Informed by their experiences with alternative payment models, physicians, practice leaders, and other market observers described ways to enhance physician practices' abilities to respond successfully. We present these as recommendations for the future and divide them into challenges and opportunities for physician practices, health plans, hospitals, EHR vendors, and regulators. Although these recommendations are based on the findings of the report, we caution that our study was not designed to assess their effectiveness empirically. Thus, these recommendations should be considered potential, not proven, solutions.

Our qualitative study was intended to describe, in detail, a broad range of ways in which alternative payment models have affected physicians and physician practices. The study was not designed to be nationally representative, however, and some of the findings described in this report could be relatively uncommon among physician practices. Therefore, to help prioritize our recommendations, we suggest that physicians, health plans, policymakers, and others first determine the applicability of our findings within the health care markets they seek to influence, either via discussions with other market participants or through more-formal research methods.

Challenges and Opportunities for Physicians and Physician Practices

We found three major changes in physician practice that were partially or completely attributed to alternative payment models: increased stress and time pressures for physicians, growth and merger of physician practices, and new types of incentives, including nonfinancial incentives, for individual physicians. Not surprisingly, we found both challenges and opportunities related to each of the changes.

Increased Stress and Time Pressure

Many respondents described increases associated with alternative payment models in the quantity and intensity of both clinical and nonclinical work for physicians, and none reported that enough existing work had been "taken off doctors' plates" to counterbalance these new tasks. New clinical tasks included consulting with other clinicians and designing workflows for patient care; these tasks were almost universally described as being worthwhile, but they could exhaust physicians. Similarly, multiple respondents reported downsides to practices' efforts to become more efficient by having physicians work to the top of license because this could increase stress and time pressure for physicians if counterbalancing changes did not also occur. Practice leaders who had, for example, hired allied health professionals to handle less intensive patient needs found that this left physicians with the most complex and difficult patient scenarios, and patient visit–scheduling systems had not yet accounted for this increase in patient intensity. At the same time, some practice leaders reported being unable to delegate certain tasks to other members of the care team because of concerns or uncertainty about state scope-of-practice laws.

New nonclinical work for physicians was almost universally disliked, especially when there was no clear link to better patient care. For example, frustration was common when physicians believed they were being asked to spend more time on documentation solely to get credit for care they had provided already. Overall, increased stress on physicians might directly harm the quality of patient care and might also serve as a marker that physicians are concerned about the quality of care they are able to provide.

There are multiple opportunities to design, test, evaluate, and disseminate the most successful strategies for accomplishing the new types of work that alternative payment models require. Related to this is the fact that, although alternative payment models can increase the nonclinical work that many physicians dread, new payment programs could also create opportunities to reallocate physician work toward more-satisfying content that could produce better, more-efficient patient care. Alternative payment models could offer a chance to rethink how physicians spend their time, and we advise getting physician input on this topic, especially regarding which activities to remove from physicians' plates (to avoid overwhelming them).

Respondents repeatedly cited a need for additional support, guidance, tools, and resources for succeeding in alternative payment models without burning out physicians and expressed appreciation when such assets were made available. Some health plans, hospitals, and professional associations have already provided such supports, noting that such capacity-building activities can increase the likelihood that alternative payment models will achieve their goals. These efforts should be encouraged and expanded.

Growth and Merger of Physician Practices

Many physician practices described growing in size and becoming affiliated with hospitals and larger organizations as attractive ways to adapt to and exert influence over alternative payment programs. However, for physicians who have concerns about loss of autonomy in larger organizations, including but not limited to changes in the physicians with whom they collaborate via referral relationships, these changes might be unwelcome. Some physicians might also encounter difficulties joining and remaining employed by large practices. Several leaders of such practices reported becoming more selective about which physicians they hired and retained; some had terminated physicians with inefficient practice patterns; and others were pessimistic about cohorts of physicians who developed their patterns of clinical practice when FFS payment was dominant (believing that these physicians would be unlikely to change in a new payment environment and hoping for a new generation to replace them). Antitrust law might also limit the extent to which physician practices can grow and merge.

To address physicians' concerns about losing autonomy, organizations that might be interested in merging, allying, or acquiring independent physician practices have an opportunity to ensure that physicians are integrated into the leadership structure of these organizations. Such an arrangement can lay the groundwork for a true working partnership between physicians and larger organizations. A wide variety of interviewees, including leaders of hospitals, health plans, and larger physician practices, reported needing such physician leadership as they transition into new payment models.

In addition, some physicians currently perceive pressures to adopt different organizational structures, often because of the varying incentives in different settings (e.g., greater FFS payment rates when a practice is hospital-owned versus independently owned). One potential opportunity is to encourage payment and regulatory policies that are, to the extent possible, setting-agnostic, creating a level playing field for the various types of organizations in which physicians practice. Although physicians might still choose to become employed by a hospital, or to join an IPA, such setting-agnostic policies would allow physicians to select an option based on the desired structure of physician practice and organization, rather than be "pushed" toward one setting or another based on regulatory and financial sustainability.

New Types of Incentives for Individual Physicians

This period of transition has also created issues related to alignment of measures and incentives faced by physician practices. For some practices, payment methods have changed just enough to result in disruptive changes to the physician workday but not enough for clear changes leading to better patient care. Some physician practices faced the "two-canoe" problem of depending on FFS and accompanying incentives for a significant portion of their revenues while working to transition to alternative payment models with potentially conflicting incentives. Many practices noted that they had little support during this transitional period and predicted ongoing need for leadership, particularly physician leadership, to navigate the transition process. For individual physicians, the two-canoe problem commonly manifested as a productivity-based financial incentive at the margin (i.e., FFS determining bonuses or even entire earnings) while being subjected to nonfinancial incentives to contain the costs of care (e.g., being asked to spend time on activities that are unpaid or poorly paid relative to the marginal FFS incentive).

Practices in risk-based payment programs noted that it was difficult to monitor physician work without using the productivity measures that typically underlie FFS payment (e.g., RVUs). However, such productivity measures create intrapractice incentives that run counter to practices' success in such alternative payment models, such as incentives to "churn patients" through the office rather than engage in potentially more-efficient, non–visit-based care. We generally found that physicians disliked being paid to do one thing while knowing their time would be better spent doing another; this sentiment was especially strongly expressed by physicians who were disappointed by the application of FFS productivity incentives to them (as individuals) even when their practices received most of their revenues through alternative payment models.

Although new financial incentives can be useful, in many instances, they frequently represent modest shares of practice revenue. In many cases, physicians reported that feedback and clear directions for practice changes were more influential than revenues received through alternative payment models. Thus, it will be important to continue to experiment and evaluate nonfinancial approaches to influencing physician behavior.

Lastly, alternative payment models offer an opportunity to identify and develop additional mechanisms of assessing and incentivizing specific physician activities, such as care coordination, care management, and alternative modalities of patient care. Respondents in multiple practices described seeking more-effective ways to reward physicians for engaging in activities important to patient care (and practice success in alternative payment models) that were insufficiently compensated by practices' current internal FFS incentives.

Challenges and Opportunities for Health Plans

Our findings point to *within-plan* challenges and opportunities that individual health plans might face as they seek to implement and operationalize alternative payment models. We also found *between-plan* challenges that emerged from interactions between the payment models, when practices contracted with multiple health plans whose payment models were dissimilar (or a single health plan applied different payment models to a practice for different patient populations).

Within-Plan Challenges and Opportunities
Operational Errors in Implementing Alternative Payment Models

The complexity and newness of some alternative payment models has led, in some instances, to operational errors—that is, failure to execute a new payment model as intended and designed. Prominent causes of these operational errors included failure to collect complete data from physician practices (or, in some instances, physician practices failing to submit data when this task was assigned to them), mistakes in specifying performance measures, inaccuracies in patient attribution, and errors in identifying which physicians worked in a given practice. The physicians and practice leaders in our sample reported viewing some of these errors as inevitable when operationalizing alternative payment models for the first time, especially because many health plans and physician practices must change billing, data management, and payment systems that have historically facilitated payment under FFS. However, persistent nonpayment of earned bonuses can dampen physicians' enthusiasm for alternative payment models, even when these models remain attractive in concept. These operational errors, although potentially minimal to health plans, can undermine trust and have large and financially meaningful ramifications for physician practices, especially those that have invested substantial time and capital in new systems to enhance patient care (in the manner the alternative payment model intended to encourage).

By proactively devising strategies to detect and correct such operational errors, health plans might help reduce the likelihood of stressing those practices that are the most eager to participate in alternative payment models. For example, health plans could conduct test runs of new alternative payment models, giving physician practices performance data, disclosing what they would have been paid if the payment model were in effect, and soliciting feedback on whether the practices detect any errors—all before actually making payments under the fully implemented new model.

Understandability of Incentives and Validity of Measures

Some physicians engaged in alternative payment models (most notably, PFP programs) reported that the changes encouraged by these new financial incentives could be unclear, even after conferring with health plan representatives. When this was the case, physicians and practice leaders were unable to devise rational responses, and any payments or penalties that transpired were perceived as being outside the practice's control, equivalent to random financial windfalls or losses. For health plans seeking to change how physician practices deliver patient care, ensuring that the purpose of new financial incentives is clearly communicated and is consistent with the payment model as implemented might enhance their effectiveness.

Similarly, unclear validity of performance measures underlying some alternative payment models (again, most notably, PFP programs) was a source of concern for some physicians and practice leaders. These concerns were most prominent when health plans developed brand-new performance measures and deployed them in a new payment model. When the fairness of these measures was unclear to physicians (e.g., when differences in performance seemed to be driven by differences between physicians' particular subspecialties or case mixes rather than by differences in how well physician practices treated their patients) or when the optimal performance score was unknown or controversial, physicians described the financial incentives associated with these measures as producing frustration rather than efforts to improve patient care. To make the best possible use of performance measures in alternative payment models, health plans should solicit input on measure validity from the physicians whose behavior they seek to influence. If even those physicians with "good" performance on a given measure express doubt about its validity (as we sometimes found in our interviews), this is a sign that the measure should be reexamined.

Supporting Practices' Data Management Efforts

We found that alternative payment models increased the importance of data management and analysis for physician practices. When performance data received from health plans were perceived as complete, timely, and accurate, physicians and practice leaders expressed appreciation for how these data enabled them to direct meaningful improvements in patient care.

Accordingly, incompleteness of data sharing by health plans, especially price data, is problematic for physician practices when alternative payment models create financial incentives to provide care more efficiently. In many cases, physicians might not have even a general sense of what items cost and certainly will not be aware of the prices in health plans' contractual arrangements with pharmaceutical companies unless health plans share price data with physician practices. If the goal of an alternative payment model is to motivate physicians to choose the most cost-efficient among clinically equivalent treatments for a given patient, failing to share the full costs of each treatment option with physician practices seems counterproductive. Put another way, alternative payment models, such as capitation and shared savings, might give health plans new opportunities to reweigh the financial benefits of receiving a price discount that prevents disclosure of pricing information (e.g., through a confidentiality clause) against the likelihood of undermining physician practices' efforts to provide more-efficient care.

In addition, some alternative payment models have required substantial new data collection and data-entry responsibilities for physician practices that involve increased time investment by physicians and allied health professionals. In such cases, health plans have opportunities to reduce or remove previous reporting requirements, such as prior authorizations, to avoid overwhelming physician practices as they respond to alternative payment models. As with disclosing previously confidential drug-price data, health plans should reconsider an economic trade-off: Are the cost savings, if any, associated with requiring prior authorizations worth the risk of causing physician burnout or preoccupying practice staff, thereby undermining physician practices' efforts to succeed in alternative payment models that encourage more-efficient care?

Because health plans often have greater experience than physician practices with collecting and analyzing data, there might be an opportunity for health plans to invest in physician practices' data infrastructure directly. There were multiple examples of health plans in this study that had provided fairly extensive support, guidance, and training in data management to physician practices that participated in alternative payment models. The perspective of these health plans was that such investments were an integral part of improving their chances of meeting long-term quality and cost goals.

Between-Plan Challenges and Opportunities
Alignment of Payment Models

In our interviews with physicians and practice leaders, we found many opportunities for greater alignment among the performance measures, financial incentives, and patient-attribution methods used by different health plans. Interviewees most prominently mentioned nonalignment among quality measures as a source of frustration (vividly described as "50 people shouting their priorities at you") that required physician practices to devote significant resources to formulating a coherent response. Similarly, when quality measures required data collection by physician practices, practice leaders found that such measures might overlap in their specifications but not be identical across health plans. Minor differences in measure specifications, by requiring practices to develop different data collection tools to capture similar data in slightly different ways, multiplied the burden of data entry and management. Therefore, efforts to harmonize such measures would likely be welcomed by most physician practices and facilitate practices' efforts to respond to any alternative payment models associated with a more streamlined measure set. To help health plans adopt a common, standard set of performance measures in a given market, it might be necessary to create limited regulatory "safe havens" that allow this type of coordination without running afoul of antitrust laws.

Challenges and Opportunities for Hospitals

In recent years, hospitals' relationships with physician practices have shifted from a vendor/purchaser relationship, in which hospitals compete with one another for the physician-driven patient revenue, to one in which hospitals now hold the balance of power in some markets both as employers of physicians in various large health systems and as important partners and allies with physician practices in others.

In alternative payment models that incentivize cost containment, especially capitation and its variants, hospitals are recast as cost centers rather than revenue generators from the perspective of health systems and physician practices at risk for costs. To hedge against potential reductions in service volume resulting from this role reversal and to better control their fates under such alternative payment models, some hospitals have acquired physician practices to become health systems that provide both inpatient and outpatient care.

These changing relationships can cause friction between physicians and hospitals, which might perceive that alternative payment models amount to a "zero-sum" game. However, to the extent that successful performance in alternative payment models depends on care coordination between inpatient and outpatient settings, these payment models also might incentivize greater cooperation and partnership between hospitals and physician practices. Additionally, hospitals and large health systems offer independent physician practices an opportunity to obtain the capital investment (especially in IT) that many need to respond effectively to data-intensive alternative payment models.

In numerous interviews, hospital and health system leaders described a critical need for physician leadership in their strategies for responding to alternative payment models. Several hospitals and health systems perceived a deficit of physician leadership and offered internal programs to help physicians develop their leadership skills.

Most prominently in episode-based and bundled payment models, interviewees in multiple institutions reported examples of physician leaders who designed care protocols that led to better, more-efficient care. But at the time of our interviews, most of these physicians had performed this work without payment or at a payment rate significantly lower than their rate for clinical care, especially for surgeons within systems that continued to pay their physicians on an FFS basis. In the long run, depending on physician volunteerism might result in suboptimal allocation of physician time to care-redesign efforts. Within hospitals and health systems, achieving better alignment between the optimal use of physician time and individual physicians' financial incentives (e.g., at least equalizing payment rates between operational redesign efforts and clinical care) could help sustain physician leadership in these efforts.

Challenges and Opportunities for Vendors of Electronic Health Record Systems

Although this study did not specifically ask questions related to EHRs, nearly every physician and practice leader we interviewed brought up the effects of EHRs, both positive and negative, on their responses to alternative payment models.

EHRs were vital to the implementation of alternative payment models that required physician practices to collect, track, and analyze clinical and administrative patient data. In addition, several physician practices developed customized decision support and order sets within their EHRs to prompt physicians and allied health professionals to follow new clinical protocols that would lead to better performance in PFP, episode-based, and capitation or shared savings models.

However, EHRs also were described as detracting significantly from physician practices' improvement efforts in multiple practices. Cumbersome EHR user interfaces, expanding physician data-entry requirements, and information overload all contributed to greater physician professional dissatisfaction, stress, and cumulative quantity of work. With new EHRs occupying so much of physicians' bandwidth for change, practice leaders reported that the looming risk of burnout constrained their ability to engage physicians more fully in efforts to respond to alternative payment models. An earlier AMA–RAND report on physician professional satisfaction described a related issue, the general frustration of physicians with EHRs, in 2013 (Friedberg, Chen, et al., 2013). Our current findings suggest that, for many physician practices, little has changed.

In addition, practices in our sample that switched EHR vendors to fulfill meaningful-use requirements found that the customized order sets and decision-support modules they had developed could not be transferred to their new EHRs. In some cases, performance in the corresponding alternative payment models suffered as a result, and the loss of these customizations was described as a setback of months to years, moving EHRs further away from their intended goal of serving as a tool for improving patient care. Finally, complex procedures for extracting data from some EHRs hindered physician practices' efforts to perform the data analyses critical to success in alternative payment models.

No practice in our sample was considering a return to paper patient records. However, improving EHR usability, enabling portability of practices' customized templates between EHR vendors (for example, via application program interfaces), and easing data extraction from EHRs all present important opportunities to improve physician practices' ability to respond to alternative payment models effectively. Vendors whose systems best support these efforts will likely find an enthusiastic audience for their products.

Challenges and Opportunities for Regulators

Our findings suggest several opportunities for policymakers to enhance the effectiveness of alternative payment models by modifying their approaches to related regulations. Some of our respondents perceived that policymakers and regulators lacked a full understanding of the pressures facing frontline physicians, leading to regulatory requirements that did not always seem to derive from a careful consideration of the needs of and demands on the time of those providing direct patient care.

Study respondents felt that financial incentives for fulfilling regulatory requirements (most prominently, meaningful use) were insufficient in the long run to cover sustainably the incurred and anticipated costs of implementation, especially for small practices. This was noted to have been an important factor leading some independent physician practices to pursue hospital ownership or affiliation with large health systems. Furthermore, the administrative challenges to implementing and reporting regulatory compliance added significant time and frustration to physicians and their practices. Finally, in some health care markets, certain policies, such as state scope-of-practice regulations related to MAs, constrained practices' ability to optimize the allocation of tasks as encouraged by alternative payment models.

To reduce the likelihood of unintended interference with the goals of alternative payment models, policymakers should carefully consider the cumulative burden on physicians and physician practices when designing new regulations. When physician practices report conflicts between regulations and optimal responses to alternative payment models, regulators have an opportunity to reconsider and revise such regulations.

Closing

The study reported here was conducted during a period of multiple simultaneous transitions for physician practices in the United States, including transitions in payment models, technology, regulations, and organizational structures. In response to these transitions, physician practices faced a challenging task: Formulate a coherent strategy that could simultaneously improve patient care, preserve or enhance physician professional satisfaction, satisfy multiple external stakeholders, and maintain economic viability as businesses.

Physicians and practice leaders were, almost universally, uncertain about the best paths forward and whether their chosen strategies would ultimately succeed. However, the effectiveness of alternative payment models ultimately depends on how physician practices, together with the patients they serve, change the provision of health care.

Our findings suggest multiple opportunities to improve the design and implementation of alternative payment models and enhance physician practices' abilities to respond to them constructively. By taking advantage of these opportunities, health plans, policymakers, and other stakeholders can enhance the effectiveness of efforts to improve the quality and efficiency of patient care.

Advisory Committee Members

- John E. Billi, M.D., professor of internal medicine and of learning health sciences at the University of Michigan Medical School, professor of health management and policy at the University of Michigan School of Public Health, and associate vice president for medical affairs of the University of Michigan
- Carolyn M. Clancy, M.D., Interim Under Secretary for Health for the U.S. Department of Veterans Affairs
- Thomas J. Curry, executive director and CEO of the Washington State Medical Association, retired
- Gerald A. Maccioli, M.D., American Anesthesiology of North Carolina
- J. James Rohack, M.D., chief health policy officer for Baylor Scott and White Health
- Susan L. Turney, M.D., CEO of the Marshfield Clinic Health System
- Richard E. Wesslund, M.B.A., founder and chair of BDC Advisors
- Nicholas Wolter, M.D., CEO of Billings Clinic.

Bibliography

Agency for Healthcare Research and Quality, "Federal PCMH Activities," undated; referenced June 1, 2014. As of February 5, 2015:
http://pcmh.ahrq.gov/page/federal-pcmh-activities

AHRQ—*See* Agency for Healthcare Research and Quality.

Alexander, G. Caleb, Jacob Kurlander, and Matthew K. Wynia, "Physicians in Retainer ('Concierge') Practice: A National Survey of Physician, Patient, and Practice Characteristics," *Journal of General Internal Medicine*, Vol. 20, No. 12, 2005, pp. 1079–1083.

American Hospital Association, *Bundled Payment*, Chicago, Ill., May 2010.

American Medical Association Center for Health Policy Research, *Socioeconomic Monitoring System*, Chicago, Ill., 1997.

Auerbach, David I., Hangsheng Liu, Peter S. Hussey, Christopher Lau, and Ateev Mehrotra, "Accountable Care Organization Formation Is Associated with Integrated Systems but Not High Medical Spending," *Health Affairs*, Vol. 32, No. 10, October 2013, pp. 1781–1788.

Beckman, Howard, Anthony L. Suchman, Kathleen Curtin, and Robert A. Greene, "Physician Reactions to Quantitative Individual Performance Reports," *American Journal of Medical Quality*, Vol. 21, No. 3, May–June 2006, pp. 192–199.

Bellafante, Ginia, "$25,000; No House Calls," *New York Times*, December 8, 2013, p. MB1.

Berenson, Robert A., and Deborah R. Kaye, "Grading a Physician's Value: The Misapplication of Performance Measurement," *New England Journal of Medicine*, Vol. 369, No. 22, November 28, 2013, pp. 2079–2081.

Berenson, Robert A., Peter J. Pronovost, and Harlan M. Krumholz, *Achieving the Potential of Health Care Performance Measures: Timely Analysis of Immediate Health Policy Issue*, Princeton, N.J.: Robert Wood Johnson Foundation, May 2013. As of February 6, 2015:
http://www.rwjf.org/en/research-publications/find-rwjf-research/2013/05/
achieving-the-potential-of-health-care-performance-measures.html

Berry, S. A., M. C. Doll, K. E. McKinley, Alfred S. Casale, and A. Bothe, Jr., "ProvenCare: Quality Improvement Model for Designing Highly Reliable Care in Cardiac Surgery," *BMJ Quality and Safety*, Vol. 18, No. 5, 2009, pp. 360–368.

Bitton, Asaf, Carina Martin, and Bruce E. Landon, "A Nationwide Survey of Patient Centered Medical Home Demonstration Projects," *Journal of General Internal Medicine*, Vol. 25, No. 6, June 2010, pp. 584–592.

Bitton, Asaf, Gregory R. Schwartz, Elizabeth E. Stewart, Daniel E. Henderson, Carol A. Keohane, David W. Bates, and Gordon D. Schiff, "Off the Hamster Wheel? Qualitative Evaluation of a Payment-Linked Patient-Centered Medical Home (PCMH) Pilot," *Milbank Quarterly*, Vol. 90, No. 3, 2012, pp. 484–515.

Bodenheimer, Thomas, Jessica H. May, Robert A. Berenson, and Jennifer Coughlan, "Can Money Buy Quality? Physician Response to Pay for Performance," Center for Studying Health System Change, Issue Brief 102, December 2005, pp. 1–4.

Bradley, Elizabeth H., Leslie A. Curry, and Kelly J. Devers, "Qualitative Data Analysis for Health Services Research: Developing Taxonomy, Themes, and Theory," *Health Services Research*, Vol. 42, No. 4, August 2007, pp. 1758–1772.

Burns, Lawton R., and Mark V. Pauly, "Accountable Care Organizations May Have Difficulty Avoiding the Failures of Integrated Delivery Networks of the 1990s," *Health Affairs*, Vol. 31, No. 11, November 2012, pp. 2407–2416.

Burton, Rachel A., Kelly J. Devers, and Robert A. Berenson, *Patient-Centered Medical Home Recognition Tools: A Comparison of Ten Surveys' Content and Operational Details*, Washington, D.C.: Urban Institute, March 1, 2012. As of February 6, 2015:
http://www.urban.org/publications/412338.html

Calsyn, Maura, and Ezekiel J. Emanuel, "Controlling Costs by Expanding the Medicare Acute Care Episode Demonstration," *JAMA Internal Medicine*, Vol. 174, No. 9, 2014, pp. 1438–1439.

Carroll, John, "How Doctors Are Paid Now, and Why It Has to Change," *Managed Care*, December 2007; retrieved May 2, 2014. As of February 5, 2015:
http://www.managedcaremag.com/archives/0712/0712.docpay.html

Casale, Alfred S., R. A. Paulus, M. J. Selna, M. C. Doll, A. E. Bothe, Jr., K. E. McKinley, S. A. Berry, D. E. Davis, R. J. Gilfillan, B. H. Hamory, and G. D. Steele, Jr., "'ProvenCare^SM': A Provider-Driven Pay-for-Performance Program for Acute Episodic Cardiac Surgical Care," *Annals of Surgery*, Vol. 246, No. 4, October 2007, pp. 613–621; discussion pp. 621–623.

Cavanaugh, Sean, "ACOs Moving Ahead," *The CMS Blog*, December 22, 2014; referenced January 4, 2015. As of February 5, 2015:
http://blog.cms.gov/2014/12/22/acos-moving-ahead/

Center for Health Information and Analysis, *Alternative Payment Methods in the Massachusetts Commercial Market: Baseline Report (2012 Data)*, Boston, Mass., December 2013.

Centers for Medicare and Medicaid Services, "Bundled Payments for Care Improvement (BPCI) Initiative: General Information," undated (a); referenced June 10, 2014. As of February 5, 2015:
http://innovation.cms.gov/initiatives/bundled-payments

———, "Linking Quality to Payment," undated (b). As of February 5, 2015:
http://www.medicare.gov/hospitalcompare/linking-quality-to-payment.html

———, "Physician Quality Reporting Initiative (PQRI) Coding and Reporting Principles," Change Request 5640, Transmittal 277, May 18, 2007. As of February 11, 2015:
http://www.cms.gov/Regulations-and-Guidance/Guidance/Transmittals/downloads/R277OTN.pdf

———, "Medicare Physician Group Practice Demonstration: Physicians Groups Continue to Improve Quality and Generate Savings Under Medicare Physician Pay-for-Performance Demonstration," Baltimore, Md., July 2011. As of February 6, 2015:
https://www.cms.gov/Medicare/Demonstration-Projects/DemoProjectsEvalRpts/downloads/PGP_Fact_Sheet.pdf

———, *Summary of 2015 Physician Value-Based Payment Modifier Policies*, c. 2014a. As of February 6, 2015:
http://www.cms.gov/Medicare/Medicare-Fee-for-Service-Payment/PhysicianFeedbackProgram/Downloads/CY2015ValueModifierPolicies.pdf

———, "Bundled Payments for Care Improvement Initiative," July 31, 2014b. As of February 6, 2015:
http://www.cms.gov/Newsroom/MediaReleaseDatabase/Fact-sheets/2014-Fact-sheets-items/2014-07-31.html

Chaix-Couturier, Carine, Isabelle Durand-Zaleski, Dominique Jolly, and Pierre Durieux, "Effects of Financial Incentives on Medical Practice: Results from a Systematic Review of the Literature and Methodological Issues," *International Journal for Quality in Health Care*, Vol. 12, No. 2, 2000, pp. 133–142.

Chernew, Michael E., Robert E. Mechanic, Bruce E. Landon, and Dana Gelb Safran, "Private-Payer Innovation in Massachusetts: The 'Alternative Quality Contract,'" *Health Affairs*, Vol. 30, No. 1, January 2011, pp. 51–61.

Christianson, Jon B., Amelia M. Bond, Emily Carrier, Peter J. Cunningham, Divya R. Samuel, and Lucy B. Stark, *Economic Downturn Strains Miami Health Care System*, Center for Studying Health System Change, Community Report 11, September 2011. As of February 8, 2015:
http://www.hschange.com/CONTENT/1244/

Christianson, Jon B., Emily Carrier, Marisa K. Dowling, Ian Hill, Ralph C. Mayrell, and Tracy Yee, *Little Rock Health Care Safety Net Stretched by Economic Downturn*, Center for Studying Health System Change, Community Report 5, January 2011. As of February 8, 2015: http://www.hschange.org/CONTENT/1181/

Christianson, Jon B., Sheila Leatherman, and Kim Sutherland, "Lessons from Evaluations of Purchaser Pay-for-Performance Programs: A Review of the Evidence," *Medical Care Research and Review*, Vol. 65, No. 6, Suppl., 2008, pp. 5S–35S.

Claffey, Thomas F., Joseph V. Agostini, Elizabeth N. Collet, Lonny Reisman, and Randall Krakauer, "Payer–Provider Collaboration in Accountable Care Reduced Use and Improved Quality in Maine Medicare Advantage Plan," *Health Affairs*, Vol. 31, No. 9, September 2012, pp. 2074–2083.

CMS—*See* Centers for Medicare and Medicaid Services.

Coffman, Janet, and Thomas G. Rundall, "The Impact of Hospitalists on the Cost and Quality of Inpatient Care in the United States: A Research Synthesis," *Medical Care Research and Review*, Vol. 62, No. 4, August 2005, pp. 379–406.

Cromwell, Jerry, Michael G. Trisolini, Gregory C. Pope, Janet B. Mitchell, and Leslie M. Greenwald, *Pay for Performance in Health Care: Methods and Approaches*, Research Triangle Park, N.C.: RTI Press, March 2011. As of February 6, 2015: http://www.rti.org/pubs/bk-0002-1103-mitchell.pdf

Damberg, Cheryl L., Melony E. Sorbero, Susan L. Lovejoy, Grant R. Martsolf, Laura Raaen, and Daniel Mandel, *Measuring Success in Health Care Value-Based Purchasing Programs: Summary and Recommendations*, Santa Monica, Calif.: RAND Corporation, RR-306/1-ASPE, 2014. As of February 6, 2015: http://www.rand.org/pubs/research_reports/RR306z1.html

De Brantes, Francois S., and B. Guy D'Andrea, "Physicians Respond to Pay-for-Performance Incentives: Larger Incentives Yield Greater Participation," *American Journal of Managed Care*, Vol. 15, No. 5, 2009, pp. 305–310.

Donelan, K., R. J. Blendon, G. D. Lundberg, D. R. Calkins, J. P. Newhouse, L. L. Leape, D. K. Remler, and H. Taylor, "The New Medical Marketplace: Physicians' Views," *Health Affairs*, Vol. 16, No. 5, September 1997, pp. 139–148.

Edwards, Samuel T., Melinda K. Abrams, Richard J. Baron, Robert A. Berenson, Eugene C. Rich, Gary E. Rosenthal, Meredith B. Rosenthal, and Bruce E. Landon, "Structuring Payment to Medical Homes After the Affordable Care Act," *Journal of General Internal Medicine*, Vol. 29, No. 10, October 2014, pp. 1410–1413.

Edwards, Samuel T., Asaf Bitton, Johan Hong, and Bruce E. Landon, "Patient-Centered Medical Home Initiatives Expanded in 2009–13: Providers, Patients, and Payment Incentives Increased," *Health Affairs*, Vol. 33, No. 10, October 2014, pp. 1823–1831.

Eijkenaar, Frank, Martin Emmert, Manfred Scheppach, and Oliver Schöffski, "Effects of Pay for Performance in Health Care: A Systematic Review of Systematic Reviews," *Health Policy*, Vol. 110, No. 2–3, May 2013, pp. 115–130.

Elmendorf, Douglas W., director, Congressional Budget Office, U.S. Congress, letter to Fred Upton, chair, Committee on Energy and Commerce, U.S. House of Representatives, about House Bill 4015, the SGR Repeal and Medicare Provider Payment Modernization Act of 2014, February 27, 2014. As of February 6, 2015: http://www.cbo.gov/sites/default/files/hr4015.pdf

Fangmeier, Joshua, "Payment Strategies: A Comparison of Episodic and Population-Based Payment Reform," Ann Arbor, Mich.: Center for Healthcare Research and Transformation, November 11, 2013. As of February 6, 2015: http://www.chrt.org/publication/payment-strategies-comparison-episodic-population-based-payment-reform/

Feder, J., Jack Hadley, and S. Zuckerman, "How Did Medicare's Prospective Payment System Affect Hospitals?" *New England Journal of Medicine*, Vol. 317, No. 14, October 1, 1987, pp. 867–873.

Felland, Laurie E., Genna R. Cohen, Paul B. Ginsburg, Elizabeth A. November, Ha T. Tu, and Tracy Yee, *Physicians Key to Health Maintenance Organization Popularity in Orange County*, Center for Studying Health System Change, Community Report 10, August 2011. As of February 8, 2015:
http://www.hschange.com/CONTENT/1226/

Fenter, Thomas C., and Sonya J. Lewis, "Pay-for-Performance Initiatives," *Journal of Managed Care Pharmacy*, Vol. 14, No. 6, Suppl. S-c, August 2008, pp. S12–S15.

FOJP Service Corporation, "The Expanding Role of Hospital Medicine and the Co-Management of Patients," *infocus*, Vol. 21, Spring 2013. As of February 6, 2015:
http://www.fojp.com/sites/fojp.com/files/InFocus_Spring13_0.pdf

Fountain, Douglas L., Joy M. Grossman, Roger S. Taylor, Effie Gournis, and Claudia Williams, "Market in Turmoil as Physician Organizations Stumble: Orange County, California," Center for Studying Health System Change, Community Report 10, Spring 1999. As of February 6, 2015:
http://www.hschange.com/CONTENT/106/

Frank, Michael, "How Your Doctor Can Improve Your Performance," *Outside*, September 11, 2014. As of February 6, 2015:
http://www.outsideonline.com/fitness/wellness/Full-Benefits.html

Friedberg, Mark W., "The Potential Impact of the Medical Home on Job Satisfaction in Primary Care: Comment on 'Patient-Centered Medical Home Characteristics and Staff Morale in Safety Net Clinics,'" *Archives of Internal Medicine*, Vol. 172, No. 1, January 9, 2012, pp. 31–32.

Friedberg, Mark W., Peggy G. Chen, Kristin R. Van Busum, Frances Aunon, Chau Pham, John Caloyeras, Soeren Mattke, Emma Pitchforth, Denise D. Quigley, Robert H. Brook, F. Jay Crosson, and Michael Tutty, *Factors Affecting Physician Professional Satisfaction and Their Implications for Patient Care, Health Systems, and Health Policy*, Santa Monica, Calif.: RAND Corporation, RR-439-AMA, 2013. As of February 6, 2015:
http://www.rand.org/pubs/research_reports/RR439.html

Friedberg, Mark W., Dana Gelb Safran, K. L. Coltin, M. Dresser, and Eric C. Schneider, "Readiness for the Patient-Centered Medical Home: Structural Capabilities of Massachusetts Primary Care Practices," *Journal of General Internal Medicine*, Vol. 24, No. 2, February 2009, pp. 162–169.

Gans, David N., "To Understand New Paymentmethods [sic], Go Back to the Future," Medical Group Management Association, c. September 2013; referenced May 2, 2014. As of February 5, 2015:
http://www.mgma.com/practice-resources/publications/mgma-connexion/2013/september-(1)/to-understand-new-payment-methods-go-back-to-the-future

Gaynor, Martin, and Robert Town, *The Impact of Hospital Consolidation: Update*, Robert Wood Johnson Foundation, Synthesis Project, Policy Brief 9, June 2012. As of February 6, 2015:
http://www.rwjf.org/en/research-publications/find-rwjf-research/2012/06/the-impact-of-hospital-consolidation.html

Gesensway, Deborah, "Capitation Still an Illusion for Many," *ACP Observer*, February 1996; referenced May 2, 2014. As of February 5, 2015:
http://www.acpinternist.org/archives/1996/02/illusion.htm

Glass, K. P., L. E. Pieper, and M. F. Berlin, "Incentive-Based Physician Compensation Models," *Journal of Ambulatory Care Management*, Vol. 22, No. 3, July 1999, pp. 36–46.

Gold, Jenny, "FAQ on ACOs: Accountable Care Organizations, Explained," *Kaiser Health News*, April 16, 2014. As of February 11, 2015:
http://kaiserhealthnews.org/news/aco-accountable-care-organization-faq/

Goldsmith, Jeff, *The Future of Medical Practice: Creating Options for Practicing Physicians to Control Their Professional Destiny*, Physicians Foundation, July 7, 2012. As of February 6, 2015:
http://www.physiciansfoundation.org/healthcare-research/the-future-of-medical-practice-creating-options-for-practicing-physicians-t/

Goroll, Allan H., Robert A. Berenson, Stephen C. Schoenbaum, and Laurence B. Gardner, "Fundamental Reform of Payment for Adult Primary Care: Comprehensive Payment for Comprehensive Care," *Journal of General Internal Medicine*, Vol. 22, No. 3, March 2007, pp. 410–415.

Grembowski, David, Cornelia M. Ulrich, David Paschane, Paula Diehr, Wayne Katon, Diane Martin, Donald L. Patrick, and Christine Velicer, "Managed Care and Primary Physician Satisfaction," *Journal of the American Board of Family Medicine*, Vol. 16, No. 5, September 1, 2003, pp. 383–393.

Grossman, Joy, Ha Tu, and Dori Cross, *Arranged Marriages: The Evolution of ACO Partnerships in California*, California HealthCare Foundation, September 2013. As of February 6, 2015: http://www.chcf.org/publications/2013/09/arranged-marriages-acos

Hackbarth, Glenn M., chair, Medicare Payment Advisory Commission, letter to Marilyn Tavenner, administrator, Centers for Medicare and Medicaid Services, about accountable care organizations, June 16, 2014. As of February 6, 2015: http://www.medpac.gov/documents/comment-letters/ comment-letter-to-cms-on-accountable-care-organizations-%28june-16-2014%29.pdf?sfvrsn=0

Halladay, J. R., S. C. Stearns, T. Wroth, L. Spragens, S. Hofstetter, S. Zimmerman, and P. D. Sloane, "Cost to Primary Care Practices of Responding to Payer Requests for Quality and Performance Data," *Annals of Family Medicine*, Vol. 7, No. 6, November–December 2009, pp. 495–503.

Havighurst, Craig, "How Physician Organizations Are Responding to Managed Care," Center for Studying Health System Change, Issue Brief 20, May 1999, pp. 1–4. As of February 6, 2015: http://www.hschange.com/CONTENT/61/?id_conf=6

Hearld, L. R., Jeffrey A. Alexander, Y. Shi, and Lawrence P. Casalino, "Pay-for-Performance and Public Reporting Program Participation and Administrative Challenges Among Small- and Medium-Sized Physician Practices," *Medical Care Research and Review*, Vol. 71, No. 3, June 2014, pp. 299–312.

Higgins, Aparna, Kristin Stewart, Kirstin Dawson, and Carmella Bocchino, "Early Lessons from Accountable Care Models in the Private Sector: Partnerships Between Health Plans and Providers," *Health Affairs*, Vol. 30, No. 9, September 2011, pp. 1718–1727.

Hill, Clara E., Sarah Knox, Barbara J. Thompson, Elizabeth Nutt Williams, Shirley A. Hess, and Nicholas Ladany, "Consensual Qualitative Research: An Update," *Journal of Counseling Psychology*, Vol. 52, No. 2, April 2005, pp. 196–205.

Horowitz, Alan S., "Should You Consider a Concierge Medicine Practice?" *The Profitable Practice*, June 28, 2013. As of February 5, 2015: http://profitable-practice.softwareadvice.com/should-you-consider-concierge-medicine-0413/

Hsiao, Chun-Ju, Esther Hing, Thomas C. Socey, and Bill Cai, "Electronic Health Record Systems and Intent to Apply for Meaningful Use Incentives Among Office-Based Physician Practices: United States, 2001–2011," Hyattsville, Md.: National Center for Health Statistics, Policy Brief 79, November 2011. As of February 6, 2015: http://www.cdc.gov/nchs/data/databriefs/db79.htm

Hussey, Peter S., Andrew W. Mulcahy, Christopher Schnyer, and Eric C. Schneider, *Closing the Quality Gap: Revisiting the State of the Science*, Vol. 1: *Bundled Payment: Effects on Health Care Spending and Quality*, Rockville, Md.: Agency for Healthcare Research and Quality, Evidence Report/Technology Assessment 208.1, Report 12-E007-EF, August 2012. As of February 6, 2015: http://www.ncbi.nlm.nih.gov/books/NBK107229/

Hussey, Peter S., M. Susan Ridgely, and Meredith B. Rosenthal, "The PROMETHEUS Bundled Payment Experiment: Slow Start Shows Problems in Implementing New Payment Models," *Health Affairs*, Vol. 30, No. 11, November 2011, pp. 2116–2124.

IHA—*See* Integrated Healthcare Association.

Integrated Healthcare Association, "IHA Overview and Principal Projects," May 7, 2014. As of February 6, 2015: http://www.iha.org/iha_principal_projects.html

Kary, Weslie, *Bundled Episode Payment and Gainsharing Demonstration*, Integrated Healthcare Association, September 2013. As of February 6, 2015: http://www.iha.org/pdfs_documents/bundled_payment/ Bundled-Episode-Payment-Gainsharing-Demo-Whitepaper.pdf

Kautter, John, Gregory C. Pope, Musetta Leung, Michael Trisolini, Walter Adamache, Kevin Smith, Diana Trebino, Jenya Kaganove, Lindsey Patterson, Olivia Berzin, and Margot Schwartz, *Evaluation of the Medicare Physician Group Practice Demonstration*, Baltimore, Md.: Centers for Medicare and Medicaid Services, Center for Medicare and Medicaid Innovation, September 2012. As of February 6, 2015: http://www.cms.gov/Medicare/Demonstration-Projects/DemoProjectsEvalRpts/Downloads/PhysicianGroupPracticeFinalReport.pdf

Keating, Nancy L., Bruce E. Landon, John Z. Ayanian, Catherine Borbas, and Edward Guadagnoli, "Practice, Clinical Management, and Financial Arrangements of Practicing Generalists: Are They Associated with Satisfaction," *Journal of General Internal Medicine*, Vol. 19, No. 5, Pt. 1, May 2004, pp. 410–418.

Kerr, E. A., R. D. Hays, B. S. Mittman, A. L. Siu, B. Leake, and Robert H. Brook, "Primary Care Physicians' Satisfaction with Quality of Care in California Capitated Medical Groups," *JAMA*, Vol. 278, No. 4, July 23–30, 1997, pp. 308–312.

Khullar, Dhruv, Robert Kocher, Patrick Conway, and Rahul Rajkumar, "How 10 Leading Health Systems Pay Their Doctors," *Healthcare*, 2014.

Kocot, S. Lawrence, Christine Dang-Vu, Ross White, and Mark McClellan, "Early Experiences with Accountable Care in Medicaid: Special Challenges, Big Opportunities," *Population Health Management*, Vol. 16, Supp. 1, 2013, pp. S4–S11.

Kolstad, Jonathan T., "Information and Quality When Motivation Is Intrinsic: Evidence from Surgeon Report Cards," *American Economic Review*, Vol. 103, No. 7, 2013, pp. 2875–2910.

Kvale, Steinar, *Interviews: An Introduction to Qualitative Research Writing*, Thousand Oaks, Calif.: Sage Publications, 1996.

Lake, Timothy K., and Robert F. St. Peter, *Payment Arrangements and Financial Incentives for Physicians*, Center for Studying Health System Change, Data Bulletin 8, Fall 1997. As of February 6, 2015: http://www.hschange.com/CONTENT/89/

Landon, Bruce E., James D. Reschovsky, A. J. O'Malley, Hoangmai H. Pham, and Jack Hadley, "The Relationship Between Physician Compensation Strategies and the Intensity of Care Delivered to Medicare Beneficiaries," *Health Services Research*, Vol. 46, No. 6, Pt. 1, December 2011, pp. 1863–1882.

Landon, Bruce E., James D. Reschovsky, Hoangmai H. Pham, Panagiota Kitsantas, Janusz Wojtuskiak, and Jack Hadley, "Creating a Parsimonious Typology of Physician Financial Incentives," *Health Services and Outcomes Research Methodology*, Vol. 9, No. 4, December 2009, pp. 213–233.

Larson, Bridget K., Aricca D. Van Citters, Sara A. Kreindler, Kathleen L. Carluzzo, Josette N. Gbemudu, Frances M. Wu, Eugene C. Nelson, Stephen M. Shortell, and Elliott S. Fisher, "Insights from Transformations Under Way at Four Brookings–Dartmouth Accountable Care Organization Pilot Sites," *Health Affairs*, Vol. 31, No. 11, November 2012, pp. 2395–2406.

Leavitt Partners Accountable Care Cooperative, "ACO Weekly Insights: 12.19.14," email newsletter, December 29, 2014.

Lewis, Sarah E., Robert S. Nocon, Hui Tang, Seo Young Park, Anusha M. Vable, Lawrence P. Casalino, Elbert S. Huang, Michael T. Quinn, Deborah L. Burnet, William Thomas Summerfelt, Jonathan M. Birnberg, and Marshall H. Chin, "Patient-Centered Medical Home Characteristics and Staff Morale in Safety Net Clinics," *Archives of Internal Medicine*, Vol. 172, No. 1, 2012, pp. 23–31.

Lewis, Valerie A., Carrie H. Colla, Kathleen L. Carluzzo, Sarah E. Kler, and Elliott S. Fisher, "Accountable Care Organizations in the United States: Market and Demographic Factors Associated with Formation," *Health Services Research*, Vol. 48, No. 6, Pt. 1, December 2013, pp. 1840–1858.

Lewis, Valerie A., Carrie H. Colla, William L. Schpero, Stephen M. Shortell, and Elliott S. Fisher, "ACO Contracting with Private and Public Payers: A Baseline Comparative Analysis," *American Journal of Managed Care*, Vol. 20, No. 12, 2014, pp. 1008–1014.

Linzer, Mark, Thomas R. Konrad, Jeffrey Douglas, Julia E. McMurray, Donald E. Pathman, Eric S. Williams, Mark D. Schwartz, Martha Gerrity, William Scheckler, JudyAnn Bigby, and Elnora Rhodes, "Managed Care, Time Pressure, and Physician Job Satisfaction: Results from the Physician Worklife Study," *Journal of General Internal Medicine*, Vol. 15, No. 7, 2000, pp. 441–450.

Lucier, D. J., N. B. Frisch, B. J. Cohen, M. Wagner, D. Salem, and David G. Fairchild, "Academic Retainer Medicine: An Innovative Business Model for Cross-Subsidizing Primary Care," *Academic Medicine*, Vol. 85, No. 6, June 2010, pp. 959–964.

Mayes, Rick, and Robert A. Berenson, *Medicare Prospective Payment and the Shaping of U.S. Health Care*, Baltimore, Md.: Johns Hopkins University Press, 2006.

McAllister, Jeanne W., W. Carl Cooley, Jeanne Van Cleave, Alexy Arauz Boudreau, and Karen Kuhlthau, "Medical Home Transformation in Pediatric Primary Care: What Drives Change?" *Annals of Family Medicine*, Vol. 11, Suppl. 1, June 2013, pp. S90–S98.

McCall, Nelda, Harriet L. Komisar, Andrew Petersons, and Stanley Moore, "Medicare Home Health Before and After the BBA," *Health Affairs*, Vol. 20, No. 3, May 2001, pp. 189–198.

McGinnis, Tricia, and David Marc Small, *Accountable Care Organizations in Medicaid: Emerging Practices to Guide Program Design*, Hamilton, N.J.: Center for Health Care Strategies, February 2012. As of February 6, 2015:
http://www.chcs.org/resource/
accountable-care-organizations-in-medicaid-emerging-practices-to-guide-program-design/

McWilliams, J. Michael, Bruce E. Landon, and Michael E. Chernew, "Changes in Health Care Spending and Quality for Medicare Beneficiaries Associated with a Commercial ACO Contract," *JAMA*, Vol. 310, No. 8, August 28, 2013, pp. 829–836.

Mechanic, Robert, P. Santos, Bruce E. Landon, and Michael E. Chernew, "Medical Group Responses to Global Payment: Early Lessons from the 'Alternative Quality Contract' in Massachusetts," *Health Affairs*, Vol. 30, No. 9, September 2011, pp. 1734–1742.

Mechanic, Robert, and Darren E. Zinner, "Many Large Medical Groups Will Need to Acquire New Skills and Tools to Be Ready for Payment Reform," *Health Affairs*, Vol. 31, No. 9, 2012, pp. 1984–1992.

Mehrotra, A., S. D. Pearson, K. L. Coltin, K. P. Kleinman, J. A. Singer, B. Rabson, and Eric C. Schneider, "The Response of Physician Groups to P4P Incentives," *American Journal of Managed Care*, Vol. 13, No. 5, May 2007, pp. 249–255.

Merritt Hawkins, "Physician Compensation, Salary and Physician Practice Surveys," undated; referenced December 10, 2014. As of February 6, 2015:
http://www.merritthawkins.com/compensation-surveys.aspx

———, "Review 2013 of Physician and Advanced Practitioner Recruiting Incentives," 2013. As of February 6, 2015:
http://www.merritthawkins.com/uploadedFiles/MerrittHawkins/Pdf/
2013_Review_of_Recruiting%20Incentives_Preview.pdf

Miller, Harold D., *Pathways for Physician Success Under Healthcare Payment and Delivery Reforms*, American Medical Association, 2010.

Morrison, Ian, "The Future of Physicians' Time," *Annals of Internal Medicine*, Vol. 132, No. 1, 2000, pp. 80–84.

Murphy, K. M., and D. B. Nash, "Nonprimary Care Physicians' Views on Office-Based Quality Incentive and Improvement Programs," *American Journal of Medical Quality*, Vol. 23, No. 6, November–December 2008, pp. 427–439.

Murray, A., J. E. Montgomery, H. Chang, William H. Rogers, T. Inui, and Dana Gelb Safran, "Doctor Discontent: A Comparison of Physician Satisfaction in Different Delivery System Settings, 1986 and 1997," *Journal of General Internal Medicine*, Vol. 16, No. 7, July 2001, pp. 452–459.

Nadler, Eric S., Suzanne Sims, Patrick H. Tyrance, Jr., David G. Fairchild, Troyen A. Brennan, and David W. Bates, "Does a Year Make a Difference? Changes in Physician Satisfaction and Perception in an Increasingly Capitated Environment," *American Journal of Medicine*, Vol. 107, No. 1, July 1999, pp. 38–44.

Nelson, K. M., C. Helfrich, H. Sun, Paul L. Hebert, Chuan-Fen Liu, E. Dolan, L. Taylor, E. Wong, C. Maynard, Susan E. Hernandez, W. Sanders, I. Randall, I. Curtis, G. Schectman, R. Stark, and Stephan D. Fihn, "Implementation of the Patient-Centered Medical Home in the Veterans Health Administration: Associations with Patient Satisfaction, Quality of Care, Staff Burnout, and Hospital and Emergency Department Use," *JAMA Internal Medicine*, Vol. 174, No. 8, August 2014, pp. 1350–1358.

Nelson, Lyle, *Lessons from Medicare's Demonstration Projects on Value-Based Payment*, Washington, D.C.: Congressional Budget Office, Working Paper 2012-02, January 2012. As of February 6, 2015: https://www.cbo.gov/sites/default/files/WP2012-02_Nelson_Medicare_VBP_Demonstrations.pdf

O'Kane, M. E., "Performance-Based Measures: The Early Results Are In," *Journal of Managed Care Pharmacy*, Vol. 13, No. 2, Suppl. B, March 2007, pp. S3–6.

Oliver Wyman, "Accountable Care Organizations Now Serve 14% of Americans," press release, New York, February 19, 2013. As of February 6, 2015: http://www.oliverwyman.com/who-we-are/press-releases/2013/accountable-care-organizations-now-serve-14--of-americans.html

O'Malley, Ann S., Grace Anglin, Amelia M. Bond, Peter J. Cunningham, Lucy B. Stark, and Tracy Yee, *Greenville and Spartanburg: Surging Hospital Employment of Physicians Poses Opportunities and Challenges*, Center for Studying Health System Change, Community Report 6, February 2011. As of February 8, 2015: http://www.hschange.org/CONTENT/1189/

O'Malley, Ann S., Rebecca Gourevitch, Kevin Draper, Amelia Bond, and Manasi A. Tirodkar, "Overcoming Challenges to Teamwork in Patient-Centered Medical Homes: A Qualitative Study," *Journal of General Internal Medicine*, Vol. 30, No. 2, February 2015, pp. 183–192.

Page, Leigh, "The Rise and Further Rise of Concierge Medicine," *BMJ*, Vol. 347, 2013, p. f6465.

Painter, Michael W., *Bundled Payment Across the U.S. Today: Status of Implementations and Operational Findings*, Newtown, Conn.: Health Care Incentives Improvement Institute, 2012. As of February 6, 2015: http://www.hci3.org/content/hci3-improving-incentives-issue-brief-bundled-payment-across-us-today

Patel, Kavita, and Steven Lieberman, "Taking Stock of Initial Year One Results for Pioneer ACOs," *Health Affairs Blog*, July 25, 2013. As of February 6, 2015: http://healthaffairs.org/blog/2013/07/25/taking-stock-of-initial-year-one-results-for-pioneer-acos/

Patel, M. S., M. J. Arron, T. A. Sinsky, E. H. Green, D. W. Baker, J. L. Bowen, and S. Day, "Estimating the Staffing Infrastructure for a Patient-Centered Medical Home," *American Journal of Managed Care*, Vol. 19, No. 6, June 2013, pp. 509–516.

Patient-Centered Primary Care Collaborative, *Proof in Practice: A Compilation of Patient-Centered Medical Home Pilot and Demonstration Projects*, January 2009.

Paustian, Michael L., Jeffrey A. Alexander, Darline K. El Reda, Chris G. Wise, Lee A. Green, and Michael D. Fetters, "Partial and Incremental PCMH Practice Transformation: Implications for Quality and Costs," *Health Services Research*, Vol. 49, No. 1, February 2014, pp. 52–74.

Peikes, Deborah N., Robert J. Reid, Timothy J. Day, Derekh D. F. Cornwell, Stacy B. Dale, Richard J. Baron, Randall S. Brown, and Rachel J. Shapiro, "Staffing Patterns of Primary Care Practices in the Comprehensive Primary Care Initiative," *Annals of Family Medicine*, Vol. 12, No. 2, March–April 2014, pp. 142–149.

Petersen, Laura A., LeChauncy D. Woodard, Tracy Urech, Christina Daw, and Supicha Sookanan, "Does Pay-for-Performance Improve the Quality of Health Care?" *Annals of Internal Medicine*, Vol. 145, No. 4, 2006, pp. 265–272.

Pham, Hoangmai H., Melissa Cohen, and Patrick H. Conway, "The Pioneer Accountable Care Organization Model: Improving Quality and Lowering Costs," *JAMA*, Vol. 312, No. 16, October 22–29, 2014, pp. 1635–1636.

Pines, J. M., J. E. Hollander, H. Lee, W. W. Everett, L. Uscher-Pines, and J. P. Metlay, "Emergency Department Operational Changes in Response to Pay-for-Performance and Antibiotic Timing in Pneumonia," *Academic Emergency Medicine*, Vol. 14, No. 6, June 2007, pp. 545–548.

Public Law 111-148, Patient Protection and Affordable Care Act, March 23, 2010. As of February 7, 2015: http://www.gpo.gov/fdsys/granule/PLAW-111publ148/PLAW-111publ148/content-detail.html

Reid, R. J., P. A. Fishman, O. Yu, T. R. Ross, J. T. Tufano, M. P. Soman, and E. B. Larson, "Patient-Centered Medical Home Demonstration: A Prospective, Quasi-Experimental, Before and After Evaluation," *American Journal of Managed Care*, Vol. 15, No. 9, 2009, pp. e71–87.

Relman, Arnold S., "Cost Control, Doctors' Ethics, and Patient Care," *Issues in Science and Technology*, Vol. 1, No. 2, 1985, pp. 103–111.

Reschovsky, James D., Jack Hadley, and Bruce E. Landon, "Effects of Compensation Methods and Physician Group Structure on Physicians' Perceived Incentives to Alter Services to Patients," *Health Services Research*, Vol. 41, No. 4, Pt. 1, August 2006, pp. 1200–1220.

Reschovsky, James D., Marie C. Reed, David Blumenthal, and Bruce Landon, "Physicians' Assessments of Their Ability to Provide High-Quality Care in a Changing Health Care System," *Medical Care*, Vol. 39, No. 3, March 2001, pp. 254–269.

Ridgely, M. Susan, David de Vries, Kevin J. Bozic, and Peter S. Hussey, "Bundled Payment Fails to Gain a Foothold in California: The Experience of the IHA Bundled Payment Demonstration," *Health Affairs*, Vol. 33, No. 8, August 2014, pp. 1345–1352.

Rittenhouse, Diane R., Lawrence P. Casalino, Robin R. Gillies, Stephen M. Shortell, and B. Lau, "Measuring the Medical Home Infrastructure in Large Medical Groups," *Health Affairs*, Vol. 27, No. 5, September–October 2008, pp. 1246–1258.

Rittenhouse, Diane R., Lawrence P. Casalino, Stephen M. Shortell, Sean R. McClellan, Robin R. Gillies, Jeffrey A. Alexander, and Melinda L. Drum, "Small and Medium-Size Physician Practices Use Few Patient-Centered Medical Home Processes," *Health Affairs*, Vol. 30, No. 8, August 2011, pp. 1575–1584.

Robinson, James C., "The End of Managed Care," *JAMA*, Vol. 285, No. 20, May 23, 2001a, pp. 2622–2628.

———, "Physician Organization in California: Crisis and Opportunity," *Health Affairs*, Vol. 20, No. 4, July 2001b, pp. 81–96.

Robinson, James C., Lawrence P. Casalino, Robin R. Gillies, Diane R. Rittenhouse, Stephen S. Shortell, and Sara Fernandes-Taylor, "Financial Incentives, Quality Improvement Programs, and the Adoption of Clinical Information Technology," *Medical Care*, Vol. 47, No. 4, April 2009, pp. 411–417.

Robinson, James C., Stephen M. Shortell, Rui Li, Lawrence P. Casalino, and Thomas Rundall, "The Alignment and Blending of Payment Incentives Within Physician Organizations," *Health Services Research*, Vol. 39, No. 5, October 2004, pp. 1589–1606.

Robinson, James C., Stephen M. Shortell, Diane R. Rittenhouse, Sara Fernandes-Taylor, Robin R. Gillies, and Lawrence P. Casalino, "Quality-Based Payment for Medical Groups and Individual Physicians," *Inquiry*, Vol. 46, No. 2, Summer 2009, pp. 172–181.

Rodriguez, Hector P., Ted von Glahn, Marc N. Elliott, William H. Rogers, and Dana Gelb Safran, "The Effect of Performance-Based Financial Incentives on Improving Patient Care Experiences: A Statewide Evaluation," *Journal of General Internal Medicine*, Vol. 24, No. 12, December 2009, pp. 1281–1288.

Rosenthal, Meredith B., Richard G. Frank, Joan L. Buchanan, and Arnold M. Epstein, "Transmission of Financial Incentives to Physicians by Intermediary Organizations in California," *Health Affairs*, Vol. 21, No. 4, July 2002, pp. 197–205.

Rosenthal, Meredith B., Z. Li, A. D. Robertson, and A. Milstein, "Impact of Financial Incentives for Prenatal Care on Birth Outcomes and Spending," *Health Services Research*, Vol. 44, No. 5, Pt. 1, October 2009, pp. 1465–1479.

Ryan, Andrew M., and Cheryl L. Damberg, "What Can the Past of Pay-for-Performance Tell Us About the Future of Value-Based Purchasing in Medicare?" *Healthcare*, Vol. 1, No. 1–2, June 2013, pp. 42–49.

Sandlot Solutions, *Swim at Your on Risk: Five Lessons for ACOs About Risk-Based Relationships*, July 2012. As of February 6, 2015:
http://www.sandlotsolutions.com/sites/default/files/documents/Sandlot-ACO-White%20Paper-July-2012.pdf

Schneider, Eric C., Peter S. Hussey, and Christopher Schnyer, *Payment Reform: Analysis of Models and Performance Measurement Implications*, Santa Monica, Calif.: RAND Corporation, TR-841-NQF, 2011. As of February 6, 2015:
http://www.rand.org/pubs/technical_reports/TR841.html

Shields, Mark C., Pankaj H. Patel, Martin Manning, and Lee Sacks, "A Model for Integrating Independent Physicians into Accountable Care Organizations," *Health Affairs*, Vol. 30, No. 1, January 2011, pp. 161–172.

Shortell, Stephen M., and Lawrence P. Casalino, "Implementing Qualifications Criteria and Technical Assistance for Accountable Care Organizations," *JAMA*, Vol. 303, No. 17, May 2010, pp. 1747–1748.

Shortell, Stephen M., Sean R. McClellan, Patricia P. Ramsay, Lawrence P. Casalino, Andrew M. Ryan, and Kennon R. Copeland, "Physician Practice Participation in Accountable Care Organizations: The Emergence of the Unicorn," *Health Services Research*, Vol. 49, No. 5, October 2014, pp. 1519–1536.

Singer, Sara, and Stephen M. Shortell, "Implementing Accountable Care Organizations: Ten Potential Mistakes and How to Learn from Them," *JAMA*, Vol. 306, No. 7, August 17, 2011, pp. 758–759.

Song, Zirui, Dana Gelb Safran, Bruce E. Landon, Mary Beth Landrum, Yulei He, Robert E. Mechanic, Matthew P. Day, and Michael E. Chernew, "The 'Alternative Quality Contract,' Based on a Global Budget, Lowered Medical Spending and Improved Quality," *Health Affairs*, Vol. 31, No. 8, July 2012, pp. 1885–1894.

Suarez, K., J. Byrne, and K. Bottles, "Physician Incentive Plan Boosts Physician/Patient Satisfaction: 5-Year-Old Plan at Priority Health Shows Success," *Physician Executive*, Vol. 29, No. 2, March–April 2003, pp. 22–25.

Sylling, Philip W., Edwin S. Wong, Chuan-Fen Liu, Susan E. Hernandez, Adam J. Batten, Christian D. Helfrich, Karin Nelson, Stephan D. Fihn, and Paul L. Hebert, "Patient-Centered Medical Home Implementation and Primary Care Provider Turnover," *Medical Care*, Vol. 52, No. 12, December 2014, pp. 1017–1022.

Teleki, S. S., Cheryl L. Damberg, Chau Pham, and S. H. Berry, "Will Financial Incentives Stimulate Quality Improvement? Reactions from Frontline Physicians," *American Journal of Medical Quality*, Vol. 21, No. 6, November–December 2006, pp. 367–374.

Tisnado, D. M., D. E. Rose-Ash, J. L. Malin, J. L. Adams, P. A. Ganz, and K. L. Kahn, "Financial Incentives for Quality in Breast Cancer Care," *American Journal of Managed Care*, Vol. 14, No. 7, July 2008, pp. 457–466.

Trude, Sally, Melanie Au, and Jon B. Christianson, "Health Plan Pay-for-Performance Strategies," *American Journal of Managed Care*, Vol. 12, No. 9, September 2006, p. 537.

Tu, Ha T., Grace Anglin, Dori A. Cross, Laurie E. Felland, Joy M. Grossman, and Lucy B. Stark, *Lansing's Dominant Hospital, Health Plan Strengthens Market Positions*, Center for Studying Health System Change, Community Report 7, March 2011. As of February 8, 2015:
http://www.hschange.org/CONTENT/1194/

Tu, Ha T., Marisa K. Dowling, Laurie E. Felland, Paul B. Ginsburg, and Ralph C. Mayrell, *State Reform Dominates Boston Health Care Market Dynamics*, Center for Studying Health System Change, Community Report 1, September 2010. As of February 8, 2015:
http://www.hschange.org/CONTENT/1145/

Ubokudom, S. E., "The Association Between the Organization of Medical Practice and Primary Care Physician Attitudes and Practice Orientations," *Social Science and Medicine*, Vol. 46, No. 1, January 1998, pp. 59–71.

Ulrich, Connie M., Karen L. Soeken, and Nancy Miller, "Ethical Conflict Associated with Managed Care: Views of Nurse Practitioners," *Nursing Research*, Vol. 52, No. 3, May–June 2003, pp. 168–175.

Ullrich, F. A., A. C. MacKinney, and K. J. Mueller, "Are Primary Care Practices Ready to Become Patient-Centered Medical Homes?" *Journal of Rural Health*, Vol. 29, No. 2, Spring 2013, pp. 180–187.

Urdapilleta, Oswaldo, Daniel Weinberg, Sarah Pedersen, Geena Kim, Stephanie Cannon-Jones, and Jenine Woodward, *Evaluation of the Medicare Acute Care Episode (ACE) Demonstration: Final Evaluation Report*, Centers for Medicare and Medicaid Services, May 31, 2013. As of February 6, 2015:
http://downloads.cms.gov/files/cmmi/ACE-EvaluationReport-Final-5-2-14.pdf

Van Herck, Pieter, Delphine De Smedt, Lieven Annemans, Roy Remmen, Meredith B. Rosenthal, and Walter Sermeus, "Systematic Review: Effects, Design Choices, and Context of Pay-for-Performance in Health Care," *BMC Health Services Research*, Vol. 10, 2010, p. 247.

Waddimba, A. C., J. F. Burgess, Jr., G. J. Young, H. B. Beckman, and M. Meterko, "Motivators and Hygiene Factors Among Physicians Responding to Explicit Incentives to Improve the Value of Care," *Quality Management in Health Care*, Vol. 22, No. 4, October–December 2013, pp. 276–292.

Wehrwein, Peter, "Pioneer ACOs: And Then There Were 23," *Managed Care*, September 2013. As of February 6, 2015:
http://www.managedcaremag.com/archives/2013/9/pioneer-acos-and-then-there-were-23

Williams, Thomas V., Alan M. Zaslavsky, and Paul D. Cleary, "Physician Experiences with, and Ratings of, Managed Care Organizations in Massachusetts," *Medical Care*, Vol. 37, No. 6, June 1999, pp. 589–600.

Wise, Christopher G., Jeffrey A. Alexander, Lee A. Green, and Genna R. Cohen, "Physician Organization–Practice Team Integration for the Advancement of Patient-Centered Care," *Journal of Ambulatory Care Management*, Vol. 35, No. 4, October–December 2012, pp. 311–322.

Wynn, Barbara O., *Medicare Payment for Hospital Outpatient Services: A Historical Review of Policy Options*, Santa Monica, Calif.: RAND Corporation, WR-267-MEDPAC, 2005. As of February 6, 2015:
http://www.rand.org/pubs/working_papers/WR267.html

Yin, Robert K., *Case Study Research: Design and Methods*, Los Angeles, Calif.: SAGE, 2014.

Zuvekas, Samuel H., and Joel W. Cohen, "Paying Physicians by Capitation: Is the Past Now Prologue?" *Health Affairs*, Vol. 29, No. 9, September 2010, pp. 1661–1666.